Emerging Challenges in Filovirus Infections

Edited by Samuel Ikwaras Okware

Published in London, United Kingdom

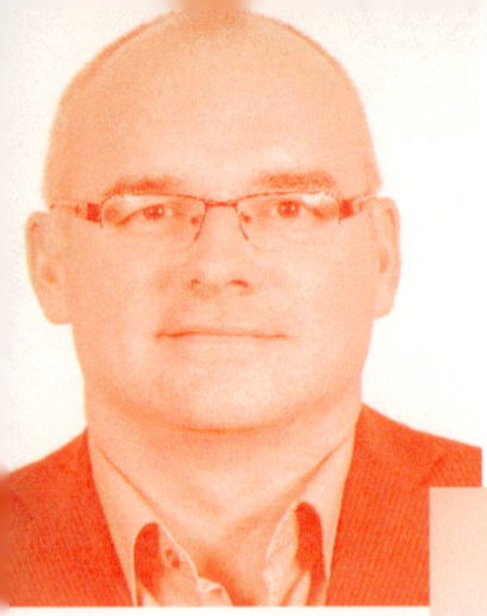
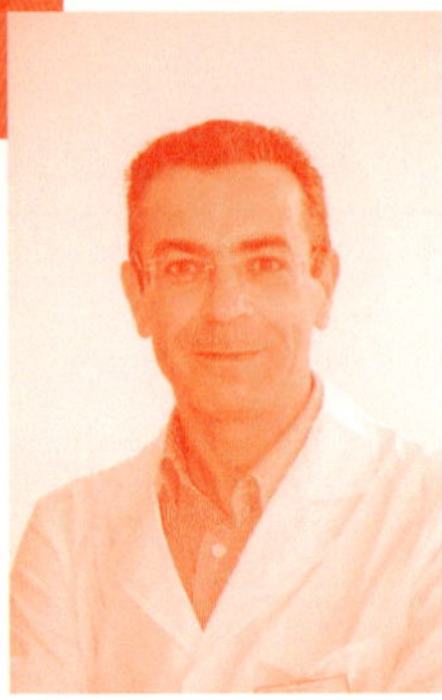
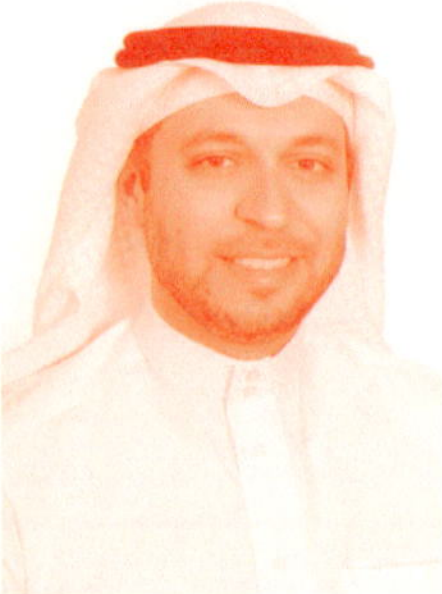
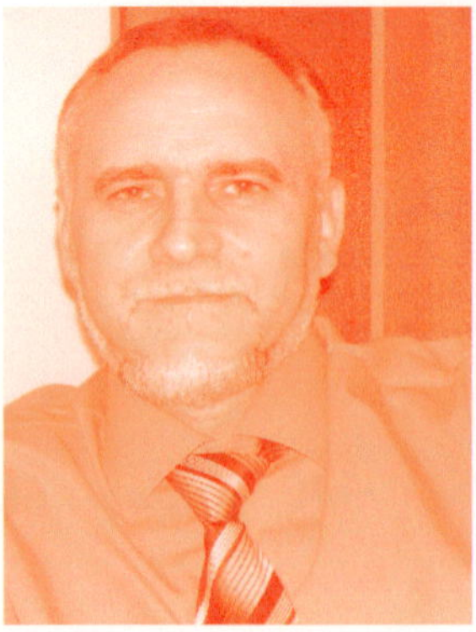
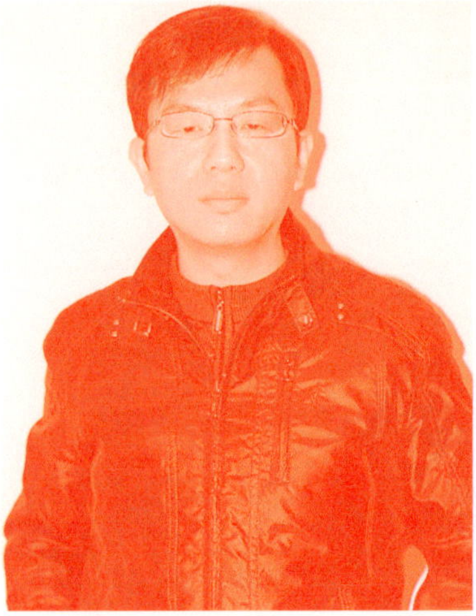
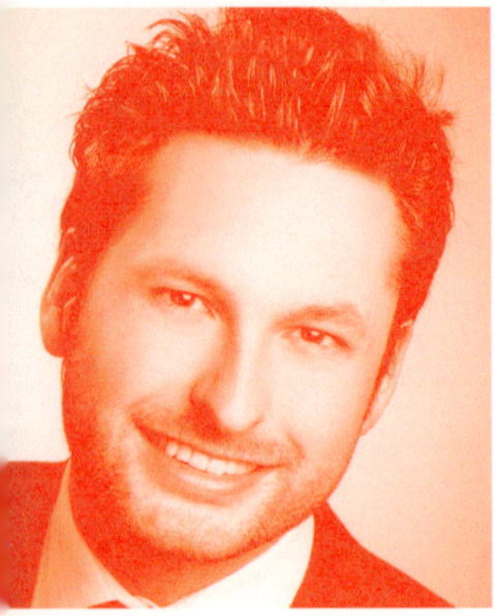
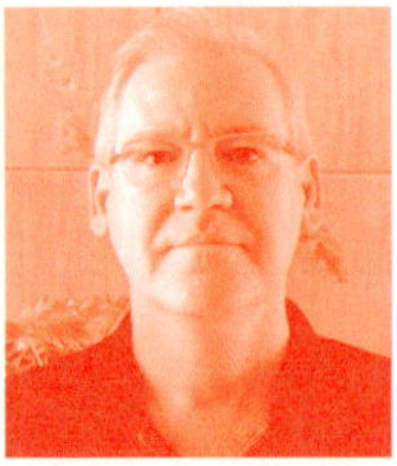

IntechOpen

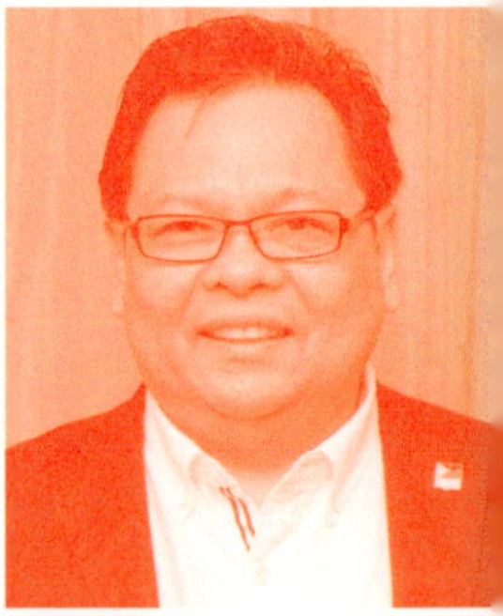
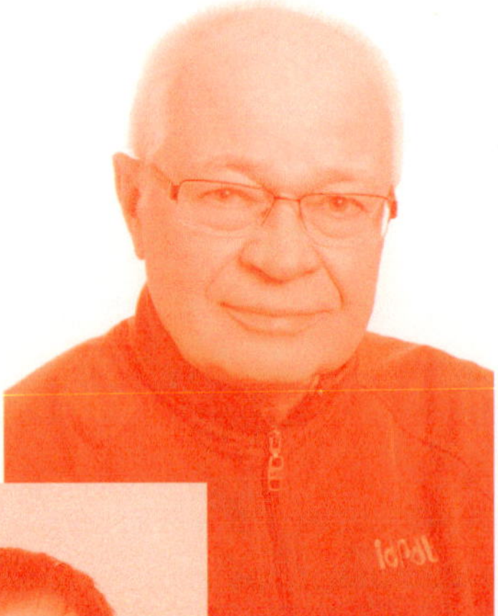
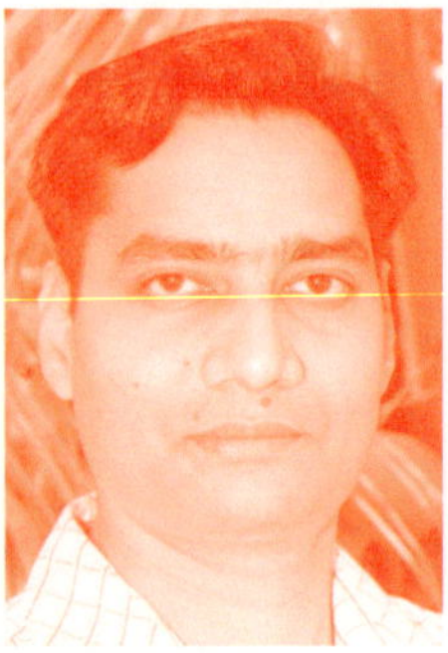
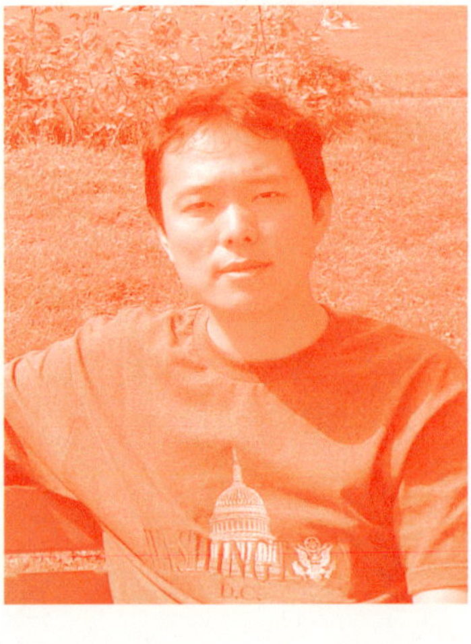
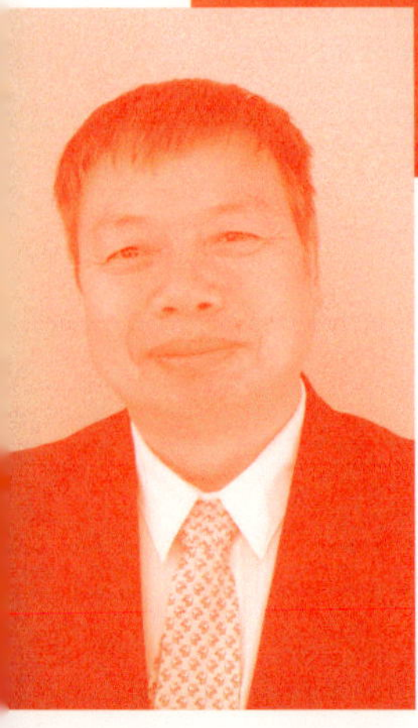
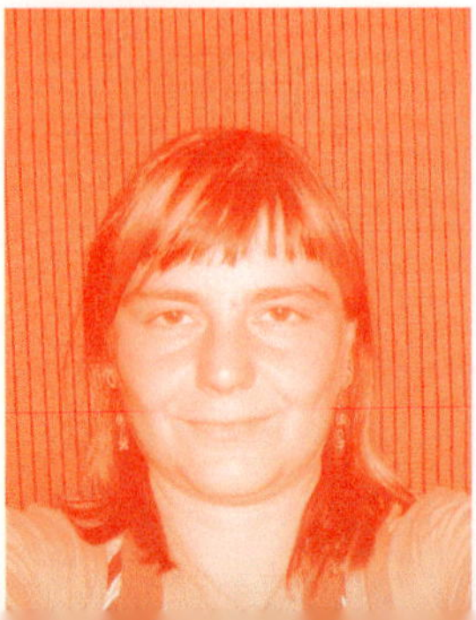

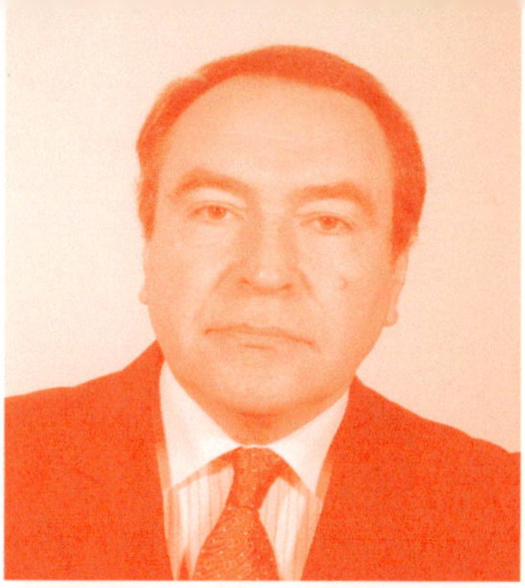

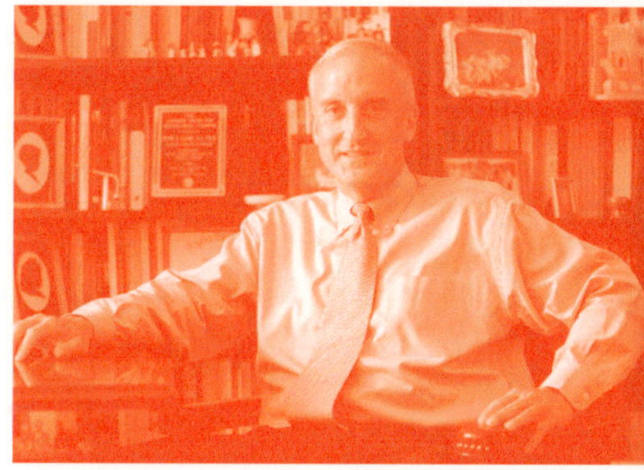

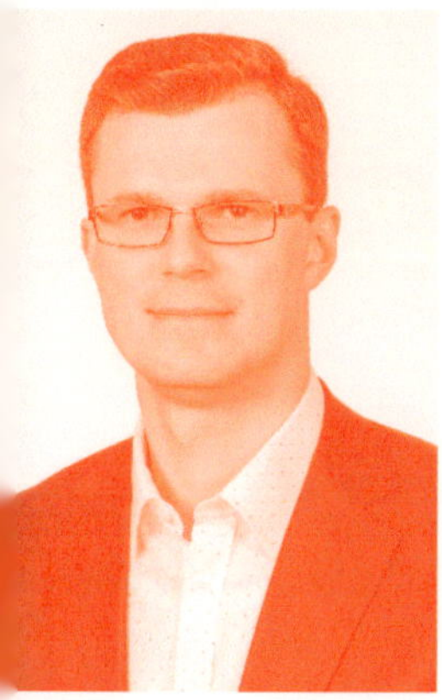

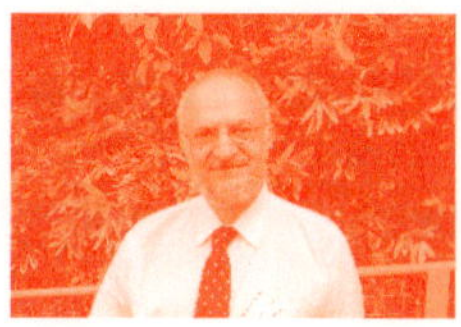

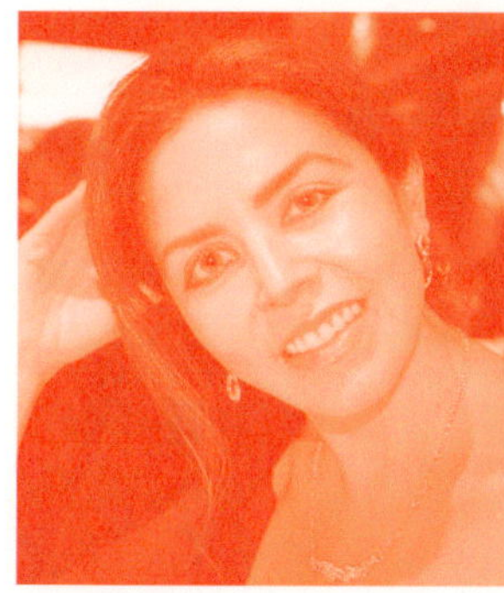

Supporting open minds since 2005

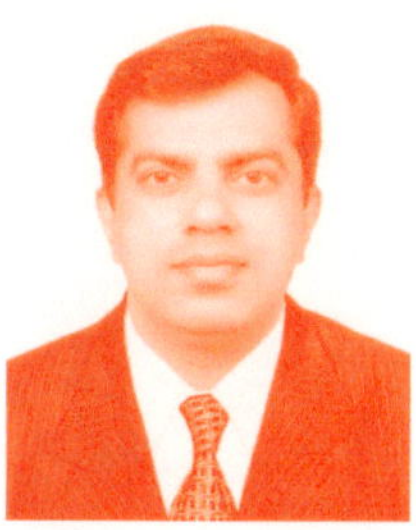

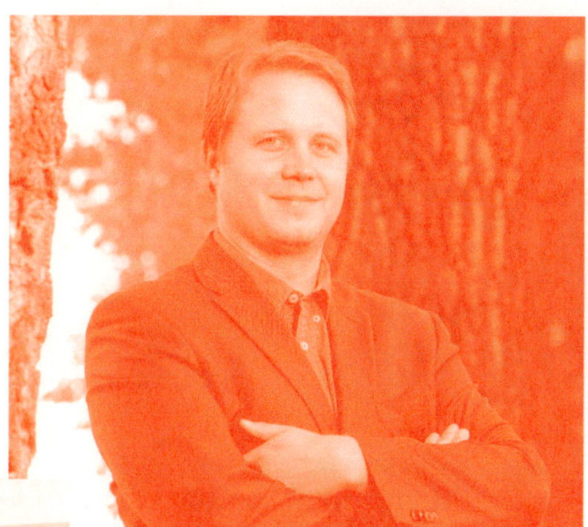

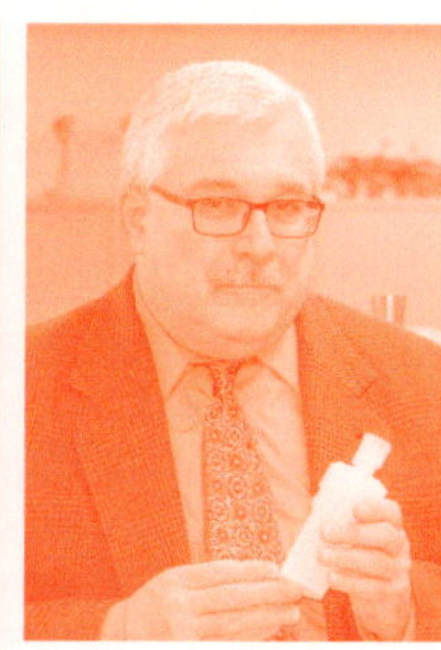

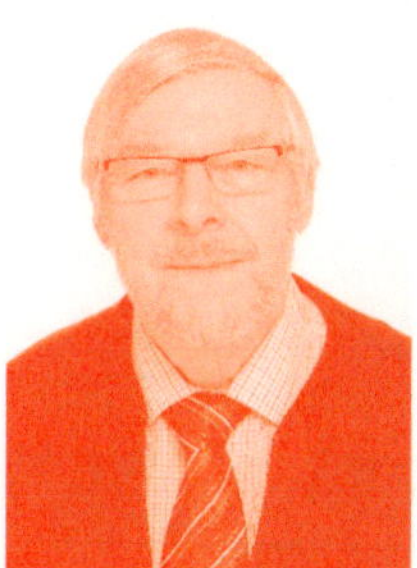

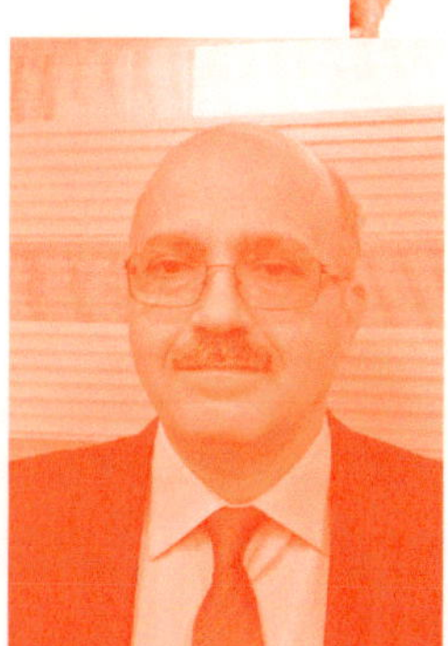

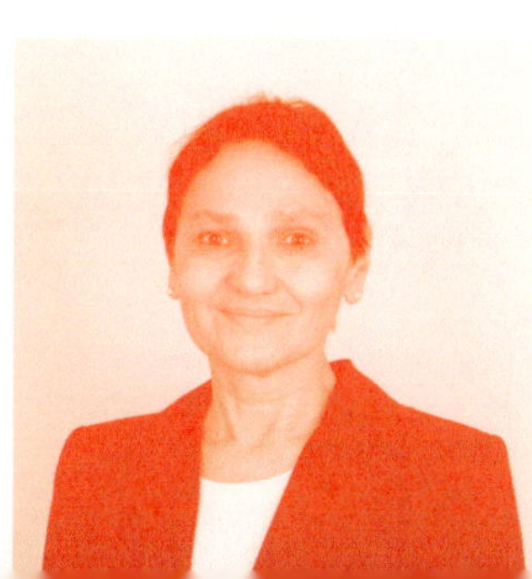

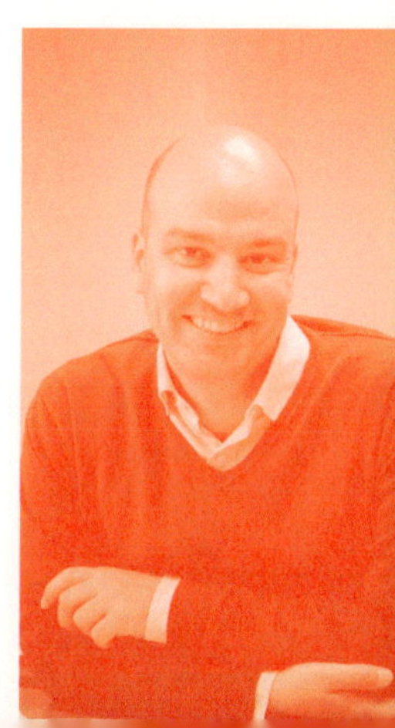

Emerging Challenges in Filovirus Infections
http://dx.doi.org/10.5772/intechopen.77719
Edited by Samuel Ikwaras Okware

Contributors
Ilkka Julkunen, Laura Kakkola, Felix B. He, Krister Melen, Manfred Weidmann, Oumar Faye, Cheikh Tidiane Diagne, Barre Soropogui, Gamou Fall, N Magassouba, Lamine Koivogui, Amadou Diallo, Sakoba Keita, Cheikh Loucoubar, Mamadou Diop, Amadou Alpha Sall, Ousmane Faye, Emily Dorothee Meyer, Cheikh Fall, Jean-Paul Gonzalez, Massamba Sylla, Tom Vincent, Marc Souris, David Schwartz, Samuel Ikwaras Okware

First published in London, United Kingdom, 2020 by IntechOpen
IntechOpen is the global imprint of INTECHOPEN LIMITED, registered in England and Wales, registration number: 11086078, 7th floor, 10 Lower Thames Street, London, EC3R 6AF, United Kingdom
Printed in Croatia

British Library Cataloguing-in-Publication Data
A catalogue record for this book is available from the British Library

Additional hard and PDF copies can be obtained from orders@intechopen.com

Emerging Challenges in Filovirus Infections
Edited by Samuel Ikwaras Okware
p. cm.
Print ISBN 978-1-78985-549-4
Online ISBN 978-1-78985-550-0
eBook (PDF) ISBN 978-1-78985-056-7

For EU product safety concerns:
IN TECH d.o.o., Prolaz Marije Krucifikse Kozulić 3, 51000 Rijeka, Croatia, info@intechopen.com or visit our website at intechopen.com.

Meet the editor

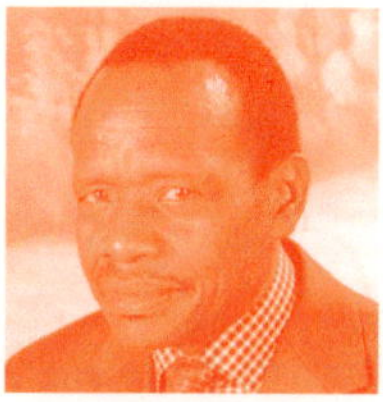

Dr Samuel Okware is a medical doctor and public health specialist with a PhD in emerging infections. He heads health research in Uganda as the Director General of the Uganda National Health Research Organization. Previously he led the containment of several major disease outbreaks of Ebola and Marburg virus diseases in Uganda. He has led pioneering research on HIV/AIDS, which contributed to one of the earliest successful HIV/AIDS Control Programs in Africa. He has supported many countries to set up national programs for AIDS control as a public health consultant. Dr Okware has international experience and was, until recently, a member of the WHO Expert Committee on Research and Development.

Contents

Preface

Filoviruses have been identified as new emerging, highly fatal pathogens. They mainly comprised the Marburg virus and the Ebola virus. There is no known cure and mortality remains very high. The Marburg virus infection was first identified in 1967 in Marburg Germany among laboratory workers who were accidentally infected by imported green monkeys. The first outbreak of Ebola virus disease occurred in 1976 in Kikwit, in the Democratic Republic of the Congo on the northern border with South Sudan. Since then several major outbreaks have occurred in Equatorial Africa, especially in the Democratic Republic of the Congo, Sudan, Angola, and Uganda. In 2014 to 2015, a major Ebola outbreak occurred in West Africa during which over 23,000 cases and nearly 10,000 deaths occurred. The outbreak spread to several countries and constituted an unprecedented global health emergency. Since then, the scientific knowledge on these pathogens has been increasing but a lot more on the ecology and treatment remains elusive.

This book discusses the emerging challenges of the filovirus infections Ebola and Marburg virus disease. It reviews the complex ecology and role of bats and other suspected intermediate hosts, including pigs. Also examined are the challenges for other modes of transmission and shortcomings in detection. The immunology and pathogenesis of the infection and the impact on the host's immune system are discussed. The rare occurrence of the Marburg infection in pregnancy and its long-term consequences of sexual spread among survivors is further examined. These discussions have the potential to support future management of outbreaks and guide research for vaccines and drugs against Ebola and Marburg disease. The book also includes historical perspectives of these viruses and discussions on the sources of major outbreaks. It also examines their complex ecology and natural habitats. The role of bats as reservoirs of infection is reviewed and evidence incriminating them as a significant source of infection is discussed. Other possible reservoirs and intermediate hosts are also examined. The challenges for the modes of spread are discussed against new scientific findings. The further discovery of the infection in pigs raises the possibility of an intermediate host or additional reservoirs. The potential for the infection to enter the food chain is examined. Evidence is also presented suggesting sexual transmission of filovirus infection with details of long-term persistence of infection in the body tissues of survivors. The book also gives an extensive review of the immunology of the infection and the impact of their interactions with the host's immune system. The pathogenesis of the diseases is analyzed. The shortcomings in procedures for early detection and diagnosis are discussed. New diagnostic tools using dried reagents adapted for field diagnosis of Ebola infection are suggested and described.

There is little information on the Marburg virus disease in pregnancy. The book describes a rare occurrence and in particular the impact of pregnancy on this infection. It also reveals the very high infectiousness and fatality rate during this period compared with known Ebola outbreaks. The role of pregnancy and the products of contraception, including the fetus, in enhancing transmission is discussed. A rare review is made of the long-term sustained sexual transmission of Marburg virus infection. Evidence for severe testicular damage and dysfunction is also reported in some detail. The discussions on the ecology, reservoirs, immunology, and the challenges in case detection have the potential to assist in the management of future outbreaks of filovirus infections as well as guide for future research agenda for related vaccines and drugs.

The editor of this book would like to thank the authors for their contributions. I also thank the Project Manager Lada Bozic for the constant valuable assistance during the preparation of this book. Many thanks also go to the IntechOpen team their support in publishing this book.

Dr Samuel Okware
Director General,
Uganda National Health Research Organisation,
Entebbe, Uganda

Section 1

Introduction

Chapter 1

Introductory Chapter: Emerging Challenges in Filovirus Control

Samuel Ikwaras Okware

1. Introduction

Infectious diseases in history have made a significant contribution to morbidity and mortality as well as disability worldwide. Nearly a quarter of the estimated 60 million reported deaths in the world each year are related to infectious diseases [1]. The influenza outbreak of 1918–1919 was the worst such incident in living memory during which nearly 40 million people died worldwide. The unprecedented *Black Death* plague outbreak in the mid 1300 equally killed millions of people. Filoviruses as emerging infections appear to be on the same path, with an ever-increasing significant global impact on public health, human traffic and commerce. The recent West African Ebola outbreak which affected 10 countries in West Africa, Europe and the USA has demonstrated its capacity to be a global threat with profound psychological, emotional and mental repercussions. Its highly virulent nature over the years and the recent West African Ebola outbreak generated considerable panic and unprecedented global public health emergency [2]. Filoviruses are comprised of the Marburg and Ebola viruses. Since the discovery of the Marburg virus disease in the 1967, and the Ebola virus disease in 1976, over 50 filovirus disease outbreaks due to *Marburgvirus and Ebolavirus* have occurred. Some 37 Ebola virus disease and 14 Marburg virus disease outbreaks occurred mostly in Africa. The recent 2013–2016 outbreak in West Africa was so far the largest and most devastating. At the end of the epidemic, about 28,000 cases and 11,000 deaths were recorded. The case fatality for both viruses is very high (34–90%). There is yet no known cure. Since July 2018, the second largest EBOV outbreak is devastating Eastern Democratic Republic of the Congo with over 1600 cases and 1000 deaths reported by October 2019 [3]. New data from the West African epidemic suggests an expansion of our understanding on ecology and geographical scope of these viruses. The pattern of occurrence and its negative impact on the economy, society and development is emerging.

2. Perspectives on ecology and transmission

Understanding the ecology and virology of filoviruses helps in designing strategies for prevention and control. Filoviruses are non-segmented negative-stranded RNA viruses. They belong to the family *Filoviridae* in the order *Mononegavirales.* There are five genera in the filovirus family: the *Marburgvirus*, *Ebolavirus*, *Cuevavirus*, *Striavirus*, and *Thamnovirus.* The Marburg virus and the Ebola virus are the most virulent to humans, while TAFV cause very limited disease and RESTV only asymptomatic infections. The *Ebolavirus* has five species known to cause disease in humans: *Zaire ebolavirus* (EBOV), *Sudan ebolavirus* (SUDV), *Tai Forest ebolavirus* (TAFV), *Reston ebolavirus* (RESTV), and the *Bundibugyo ebolavirus* (BDBV). In addition the *Bombali ebolavirus* was recently discovered in fruit bats in

Sierra Leone and Kenya. Also a new distinct filovirus, the *Dianlovirus* genus, has been proposed following the recent discovery of the *Měnglà virus* (MLAV) in fruit bats in China [4], demonstrating further the expanding geographical scope of the Ebola virus ecology. It is yet to be fully determined whether the impact of population pressures such as deforestation and forest encroachment or subsequent climate change has also leveraged the ecosystems for transmission.

The origin of the infection and its life cycle is partly elusive. It is generally accepted that the infection is a zoonosis linked to wildlife reservoirs principally fruit bats and non-human primates. Studies indicate that such bats may be the ultimate reservoirs of this infection. Epizootics in wildlife have also been reported prior to outbreaks. It is also suggested that in endemic countries, non-human primates and other animals including pigs, dogs, duikers and even arthropods may be involved in the cycle linking wildlife infection to humans [5]. Direct contact during hunting and eating bush meat facilitates rapid spread. At community level, funeral ceremonies of the victims amplify further transmission. In reported outbreaks of Marburg virus infection in Kenya, Angola, the Congo Republic and the DRC, Uganda has demonstrated cave-dwelling fruit bats as the source of infection. Serological ecological studies also have showed sero-positivity in asymptomatic individuals in selected communities in the DRC. Among the pigmy population nearest to the forest, the sero-positivity for EBOV is high and nearly 10-fold. Sexual transmission of Ebola infection among survivors raises concerns. Questions remain on the role linking these observations particularly the role of asymptomatic individuals in the community outbreak initiation.

3. Challenges on case detection

The clinical features of Ebola virus disease and Marburg virus disease have been consistent and the basis for the case definition in the detection of cases and contact tracing. The clinical features are typically high-grade fever associated with severe bleeding tendencies and followed by a rapid descent to multiple organ failure, shock and death within days. However these symptoms are nonspecific and mimic several many tropical conditions such as malaria which is so endemic and responsible for up to a quarter of the patient load in typical low-resource settings. This may undermine the timely detection of cases in outbreak management and affect the implementation of contact tracing using the WHO syndrome based on the case definition and criteria. The WHO has outlined the case definition criteria of an *alert* case, a *suspected* case, a *probable* case and a *confirmed* case. The first three are based on clinical symptom assessment, and only the confirmed case depends on laboratory confirmation with RT-PCR or IgG antibody and virus antigen for Ebola virus and Marburg virus. However, the specificity and the positive predictive values in reported laboratory tests have not been accurately determined. The challenge in making a diagnosis is that the positive predictive value of the criteria may differ from outbreak to outbreak. Studies are therefore needed for concurrent validation of the case definition at localised field conditions and identification of cross-reactions in asymptomatic individuals. Concurrent validation studies should be carried out during outbreak management and containment. Therefore the search for new and accurate diagnostic methods needs to be addressed.

The factors behind the emergence of new pathogens are complex but are facilitated partly by the enabling interaction between the host and the agent in the supported by conducive environmental factors. Apparently for emerging infections, pathogens evolve and create new phenotypic properties that adapt infectious agents to new or old hosts. The genetic variation may lead to increased virulence and infectivity. Understanding these factors including the immunology and the interactions between the filovirus and the host immune system is critical. Such knowledge will support the development of better diagnostics and tools. These tools will facilitate surveillance and outbreak management. It will provide evidence for the development of effective drugs and vaccines against the infection.

This book reviews and discusses known filovirus outbreak experiences. In particular, it examines opportunities and the missing links in the ecology, the natural history, immunology and the interactions with the host innate immune systems and other infections. It examines the potential benefits that would shape future research priorities. Such efforts could lead to quality and timely outbreak detection. Early detection and early action appear to be best approach, but such strategies should use evidence for prevention and control.

4. Conclusion

The epidemiology and the ecology together with the life cycle remain elusive. Studies are required to improve early detection to facilitate quick action. The unpredictability of the outbreaks suggests that basic epidemiological research for prevention and control should be carried out before, during and after outbreaks. Understanding the gaps in the ecology and the natural cycles of the filoviruses as well as its reservoirs will lead to the development of better strategies for prevention, control and management of future outbreaks. Campaigns directed at communities and tourists would be of benefit. Studies are needed to improve future forecasting of outbreaks. The impact of these viruses on the economy and society in general is an important area for future research. There is therefore a need for a strong global strategy that ensures international and interagency collaboration. International efforts are required to coordinate research to develop preventive strategies and tools. Support is required to support national efforts to build health systems for surveillance and emergency disease preparedness. A Global Health framework for coordination and financing of research into emerging infections will support and facilitate containment at national and global levels. The chapters in this book have tried to discuss some of these challenges and made suggestions for future research.

Author details

Samuel Ikwaras Okware
Uganda National Health Research Organisation, Entebbe, Uganda

*Address all correspondence to: okwares@gmail.com

References

[1] Fauci AS, Touchette NA, Folkers GK. Emerging infectious diseases: A 10-year perspective from the national institute of allergy and infectious diseases. Emerging Infectious Diseases. 2005;**11**:519-525

[2] Centers for Disease Control and Prevention. 2014-2016 Ebola Outbreak in West Africa. 2018. Available from: https://www.cdc.gov/vhf/ebola/history/2014-2016-outbreak/index.html [Accessed: 9 July 2019]

[3] Centers for Disease Control and Prevention. Ebola Outbreak in eastern Democratic Republic of Congo Tops 1000 cases. CDC Newsroom. 2019. Available from: https://www.cdc.gov/media/releases/2019/s0322-ebola-congo.html [Accessed: 16 April 2019]

[4] Yang X-L, Tan CW, Anderson DE, et al. Characterization of a filovirus (*Měnglà virus*) from Rousettus bats in China. Nature Microbiology. 2019;**4**:390-395

[5] Leroy EM, Rouquet P, Formenty P, et al. Multiple Ebola virus transmission events and rapid decline of central African wildlife. Science. 2004;**303**:387-390

Section 2

Ecology

Chapter 2

Essay on the Elusive Natural History of Ebola Viruses

Jean-Paul Gonzalez, Marc Souris, Massamba Sylla, Francisco Veas and Tom Vincent

Abstract

This chapter presents a review of what is known about the natural history of the Ebolaviruses in Central and West Africa as well as in the Philippines. All the previous hypotheses on the natural cycle of Ebolavirus are revisited. Also, the main factors driving the virus natural cycle are summarized for the different ecosystems where the Ebolavirus is known to have emerged, including the virus species, the date of emergence, the seasonality, the environmental features, as well as the potential risk and associated factors of emergence. The proposed hypothesis of the Ebolavirus natural cycle prevails an inter-species spillover involving several vertebrate hosts, as well as biotic and abiotic changing environmental factors among other original features of a complex natural cycle. It is also compared with other virus having such type of cycle involving chiropteran as potential reservoir and vector and presenting such original inter-outbreak epidemiological silences. Ultimately, these observations and hypotheses on Ebolavirus natural cycles give some insight into the potential drivers of virus emergence, host co-evolution, and a spatiotemporal dimension of risk leading to identify high risk areas for preventing emerging events and be prepared for an early response.

Keywords: Ebolavirus, bats, chorology, natural cycle, host, one health

1. Introduction

It has been several decades since an unknown fever dramatically emerged, close to the Ebola river, a small tributary of the great Ubangi river in the heart of the Congolese tropical forest of Africa. Since that time, even though the virus responsible for this new hemorrhagic fever has been identified and characterized, the natural history of the eponymic Ebolavirus remains largely unknown. The cradle of the virus remains enigmatic and the emergence of the Ebola fever unsolved. Indeed, the arcane of Ebolavirus natural history is still hypothesized, thanks to an elusive virus that always risen where it was not expected, violent and devastating, and surprising local populations and health systems, as well as the international scientific community. This Ebolavirus eco-epidemiology remains complex while the Ebola fever (alias Ebolavirus Disease) can be considered as an exemplary disease that can be eventually comprehended only with a trans-disciplinary approach that has recently been promoted as a One Health concept. Indeed, it is only when we take into account all disease and virus drivers, including biotic and abiotic factors of the natural and human environments, that some mechanisms of the Ebolavirus disease emergence, such as spread and circulation, can be ultimately unveiled. For that, we have collected all information available, often estimated, from the time and place of the virus emergence long before the emerging event was identified as it and the epidemic phase was brought to public attention. Moreover, when available we also collect all data on potential natural and accidental hosts, weather and environment chorology, among other multiple factors potentially involved.

Historically, Ebolavirus emerged in Central Africa in the late 1970s, and has re-emerged most recently with the active epidemic (April 2019) in the eastern Democratic Republic of Congo (DRC), by encompassing more than 24 epidemic events from Central to West Africa, to imported infected monkey from Asia to Virginia, and the emerging new Ebola species of the Philippines archipelago [1].

Among the negative sense RNA viruses of the *Filoviridae* family five genera are known, including *Cuevavirus, Ebolavirus, Marburgvirus*, *Thamnovirus*. Among the *Ebolavirus* genus, five Ebolavirus (EBOV) species have been identified [2].

Ebolavirus' (EBOV) first emergence occurred in 1976, as two different EBOV species in two different places in sub Saharan Africa. The Zaire Ebolavirus (ZEBOV) species and the Sudan Ebolavirus (SUDV) were detected concomitantly, a few weeks apart, respectively in the Northeastern Equator province of the Democratic Republic of Congo, DRC (alias Zaire), and in the Bahr el Ghazal province of South Sudan. On the 26th of August 1976 ZEBOV was isolated from missionaries and local villagers of the Yambuku, in the rain forest close to the Ebola river. However, earlier in June 1976, the SUDV had broken out among cotton factory workers in Nzara, Sudan (now in South Sudan) [3].

Then, in 1989, the Reston Ebolavirus species surprisingly (RESTV) emerged in the US (!) and was identified during an outbreak of simian hemorrhagic fever virus in crab-eating macaques from Hazleton Laboratories (now Covance) of Reston county, Virginia. Such primate specimens were found to be recently imported from the Philippines. Then, in 1994 a fourth new species of Ebolavirus was isolated from chimpanzee leaving in the Tai Forest of Côte d'Ivoire and named Côte d'Ivoire ebolavirus (CIEBOV). Finally, in November 2007, a fifth Ebolavirus species, was detected from infected patients in Uganda in the Bundibugyo District and was subsequently identified by the eponymic name of Bundibugyo Ebolavirus [4].

Briefly and extraordinarily among the world of the viruses, the filovirus virion presents a bacilliform (filamentous) shape, like a Rhabdovirus, but presents unique pleomorphic figures with branches and other tortuous shapes. Ebolaviruses have also an unusual and variable long length - up to 805 nanometers (only some plant virus can compete to this filamentous extensive length). However, the internal structure is more classical with a ribonucleoprotein nucleocapsid, a lipid envelope and seven nanometers size spikes. The genome is non-segmented, single stranded RNA of negative polarity with lengths of about 18.9 kb that code for seven proteins, each one having a specific function [5].

Ebolaviruses are known for their high case-fatality rate (CFR) with always less than 2/3 of survivors among the identified cases. ZEBOV, the most frequently isolated Ebolavirus species during the outbreaks, has the highest CFR, up to 90% in some instances, with an average of 83% for the past 37 years. The Uganda BDBV outbreak had a mortality rate of 34%. RESTV imported to the US did not cause disease in exposed human laboratory workers. The scientist performing the necropsies on CIEBOV infected chimpanzees got infected and developed a Dengue-like fever, fully recovered 6 weeks after the infection while treated in Switzerland.

2. When Ebolavirus raised his head in the heart of darkness

Dates and time make History. Indeed, the various reports on the emergence of Ebolavirus in Africa show discrepancies and lack accuracy, for multiple reasons (remote event, reports by different person or team, at different time...) but the only way to forge the history is to label the events with date, time and the environmental factors observed. On July 27, 1976, the first (known) victim to contract Ebolavirus was a cotton factory worker from Nzara, Sudan. Then, in Zaire (DRC) on September 1, 1976, the first Ebolavirus (Zaire ebolavirus, ZEBOV) victim was a teacher who had just returned from a family visit to northern Zaire (6 Jennifer Rosenberg Internet). These two events were the very beginning of the boundless journey of a deadly Ebolavirus outbreaks.

2.1 The Ebolavirus species emerging events

When the virus becomes epidemic in a human population, it does so weeks or months after the emergent event of the virus switching from its silent transmission in a natural cycle to a zoonotic/epidemic manifestation, revealed to the local health system. Let us see in more detail such emerging events of Ebolavirus species (ICTV, 2018) as there were reported or sometime interpreted, in time and place.

Sudan ebolavirus (SEBOV) occurred when the first recorded SUDV broke out among cotton factory workers in Nzara, South Sudan in June 271,976. This was indeed, the first case of Ebolavirus infection recorded and confirmed and also reported as potentially exposed to chiropteran. Indeed, at the Nzara Cotton Manufacturing Factory this first patient was a cloth room worker where bats (mostly *Tadarida* - mops - *trevori*) have a large population in the roof space of their premises. He died in the Nzara hospital on July 6, 1976. Local animals and insects were tested for Ebolavirus without success [6, 7].

Zaire ebolavirus (ZEBOV) was reported in the Mongala district of the Democratic Republic of Congo (DRC; alias Zaire) in August 1976, when a 44-year-old schoolteacher of the Yambuku village, became the first recorded case of Ebolavirus infection in DRC. Also, the schoolteacher travel earlier in August 1976 near the Central African Republic border and along the Ebola River, estimated 90 km NW from the village [6].

Reston ebolavirus (REBOV) had its first emerging event as an imported infected cynomolgus monkey (*Macaca fascicularis*) in October 1989 imported from a facility in the Philippines (Mindanao Island) to Reston, Virginia, USA, where the primate got sick and the virus isolated [8]. In the Philippines, in several instances, the virus was found to infect pigs, in June and September 2008 ill pigs were confirmed to be infested by REBOV (Ecija and Bulacan, Manila island), as well during 2008–2009 epizootics in the island of Luzon (Philippines) [9].

Cote d'Ivoire ebolavirus (CIEBOV) was isolated for the first time, and as an only known appearance, in November 1994, from wild chimpanzees presenting severe internal bleeding of the Taï Forest in Côte d'Ivoire, Africa. A researcher became infected when practicing a necropsy on one of these primates, he developed a dengue syndrome and survived. At that time, many dead chimpanzees were discovered and tested positive for Ebolavirus. However, the source of the virus was believed to be of infected western red colobus monkeys (*Piliocolobus badius*) upon which the chimpanzees preyed [10].

Bundibugyo ebolavirus (BDBV) was then discovered during an outbreak of Ebolavirus in the Bundibugyo District (Bundibugyo and Kikyo townships), on August 1st, 2007, in Western Uganda (Towner et al. [11]). BDBV second emerging event was observed in the DRC in August 17, 2012 in Isiro, Pawa and Dungu, districts of the Province Orientale [11].

With the exception of REBOV in Philippines and CIEBOV in West Africa, all other EBOVs species emerged in the Central African region. Also, all EBOVs are known to emerged in the tropical rain forest during the inter-season between dry and rainy seasons. Also, REBOV appears to actively circulate in the tropical rain or moist deciduous forest of the Philippines [12].

2.2 From Central Africa to West Africa

2.2.1 Concurrent emergences of Ebolaviruses

On several occasions, concurrent emerging events of Ebolavirus have been observed. Indeed, such events occurred in places geographically distant, independent, and unconnected. The Ebolavirus was isolated and the strains different, even they belonged to the same species of Ebolavirus, altogether in favor of a different origin from an elusive natural reservoir, thus eliminating the notion of leaping from one site to the other. In that matter, the following observations are a paradigm: From its inceptive emergence the Ebolavirus was identified in Sudan at the cotton factory and a few days later at Yambuku, Zaire. The Ebola Sudan and Ebola Zaire viruses emerged concurrently in 1976 in the Congo basin of Central Africa; More than 20 years later the virus emerged and reemergence from 1994 to 1996 in a different places in Gabon, in a successive and timely overlapping events but in unconnected areas from where different strains of the same EBOVZ were isolated [13]; More recently, during the 2014–2016 dramatic Ebolavirus disease (EVD) emergence of in West Africa where the virus emerged in late December 2013 of a 18-month-old boy from the small village of Meliandou (Guéckédou district, South-Eastern Guinea) believed to have been infected by bats [14], concurrently, in August 2013, the Ebolavirus reemerged in the Equator province of DRC - different places and different strain of ZEBOV [15].

It is remarkable that most of these emerging events occurred during or close to the end of the rainy season which generally stretches from August to October in the domain of the Congo basin tropical rain forest.

Altogether, these observations are in favor of environmental factors of emergence favoring, when they occur synchronously in the same place, the spillover of the virus from its hidden natural cycle to an accidental and susceptible host. Therefore, these plural and concomitant emerging events play against the theory of Ebola virus diffusing in oil spot in Central Africa [16]. This original pattern of concurrent emergences could explain also the relative stability of the virus strains which remain for years in the same environment, and the interepidemic silences which require several fundamentals (i.e. concurrent risk factors) to be broken.

2.2.2 An unexpected broader domain of Ebolavirus circulation

The first evidence that showed that Ebola virus had previously circulated in areas without any known cases of disease came in 1977, near the Ebola outbreak in Tandala, DRC, just 200 miles west of the first known cases in 1976 [17]. Blood samples obtained from individuals in areas with no previous symptoms of Ebola were found to contain antibodies for Ebolavirus, indicating a previous or ongoing infection with that virus. Because subclinical illness is always a possibility with viral infections, the presence of these Ebolavirus-specific antibodies could only be explained by exposure to the virus, which is somewhat reasonable in an area that is endemic to the disease. But how do we know the true endemic zone of a virus such as Ebolavirus?

Endemic zones are primarily based on where disease can most likely be expected, and are determined by historical accounts of disease, as well as supplemental information such as where animals or insects that might transmit the disease are located. With respect to the Ebola virus, outbreaks that occur in Central Africa, in or near the Congo River Basin, are expected; outbreaks that take place elsewhere are unexpected and can be problematic, as was the case for the 2014–2016 West African outbreak. And yet, scientists have highlighted the presence of Ebola antibodies well outside the endemic zone for disease for decades.

In the early 1980's, research based at the Pasteur Institute in Bangui, Central African Republic, demonstrated for the first time that the population of central Africa presented natural antibodies against the Ebolavirus strains of Zaire and Sudan [3, 4]. Research also showed for the first time that several mammal species had Ebolavirus-reacting antibodies, including rodents, dogs, and others. Initially, the scientific community was skeptical of the findings, due to the type of antibody tests used, and because the prevalence of these antibodies was unbelievably dispersed and at a high level of prevalence. However, a 1989 follow-up study confirmed methodology and preliminary observations, and expanded the results to include similar observations in Cameroon, Chad, Gabon, and Republic of Congo (the latter two of these countries would have their first Ebola outbreaks in 1994 and 2001, respectively) [5]. Moreover, such Ebolavirus antibody prevalence was found in West Africa (e.g. Senegal, Chad, Sierra Leone), preceding the catastrophic 2014–2016 Ebolavirus outbreak [18]. Subsequent studies have determined that 20–25% of persons living in or near the Congolese rain forest are seropositive for Ebola, despite never exhibiting symptoms [19].

Today, Ebola antibody prevalence is widely distributed across the African continent in the absence of severe clinical presentation and/or outbreak manifestation. A 1989 study even found Ebola Zaire antibodies among people living in Madagascar, an island country that has never had a single known case of Ebola, and which has been geographically separated from continental Africa for 100 million years [20].

Risk mapping, including ecological and geographical distribution <10-13 cm/s first hour, and extended, highly sensitive and specific environmental and biogeographical models based on EBOVs susceptible mammalian biogeography in Africa, show a robust and precise potential distribution of EBOVs in Africa that clearly overlap the African tropical rain forest biome of the Guinea-Congo forests (including the Congo basin rain forest, and the Occidental relic of the Congolese rain forest spreading from Guinea to Ghana) and the southern band of the Sudan-Guinea Savanna [21].

Also, as a result of potential Ebolavirus (or Ebolavirus antigen) exposure, serological markers have been found in vertebrates outside of Africa. With the exception of Philippines, where REBOV is known to circulate in monkeys and pigs, thus showing its ability to infect multiple animal species, in several instances serological evidence of Ebolavirus exposure has been detected in many vertebrates, particularly chiropterans [9]. Definitely, bat populations in Bangladesh and China present antibodies against ZEBOV and REBOV proteins [22, 23]. Ultimately, it appears that EBOVs are widely distributed throughout Africa, West and Central, and Asia. Moreover, risk mapping of filovirus ecologic niches suggests potential areas of EBOVs distribution in Southeast Asia [24].

The unexpected detection of REBOV first in Virginia, for the reason we know, and then the astonishing discovery of its circulation and natural cycle in the Philippines gave a rethinking of the entire family of Ebola viruses previously known mainly on the African continent [25].

From these observation and facts, the potential circulation of EBOVs in its natural cycle appears much wider than expected, while the emerging events we can witness appears to be only a tip of the iceberg in the wide Congolese tropical rain forest.

2.3 From the index case to the epidemic chain, outbreak, and pandemic

The fundamentals of emergence are changing in the heart of the rainforest and elsewhere: changing times, when the means of transmission switch from foot to motorbike, when knowledge conveyance has switched from paper reporting to the internet.

Let us examine the risk of expansion for Ebolavirus. Indeed, the factors of transmission of the virus to man and man to man are essential to take into account in this context. Moreover, it is extremely important to note that these factors are subject to permanent changes in societies whose trade and means of communication are drastically changing as a result of health systems, responses and preparedness for epidemics at national and international levels, policies, and the economy.

So, with the experience gained for more than 40 years, the strategies of struggle are clearly defined, but the societal changes that are taking place make their application difficult and sometimes impossible (e.g., the 2019 outbreak in the DRC, where political institutions have prevented an adapted response). Situation and the epidemic are perpetuated.

There is also a growing means of communication, both smartphones and motorized transport, to travel more quickly as ever, between the epidemic zone of EVD and the family [26].

Thus, during the emergence of the Ebola virus in West Africa, all of this means of communication played a fundamental role in the regional spread of the epidemic, until it became a pandemic risk when the virus was exported to other countries of the African continent and, outside Africa in Europe and North America [27].

3. A strange iteration of epidemic events with unexplained virus disappearance

It is known for several other transmitted viruses that during the inter-epidemic silences several factors can be responsible. In general mass herd immunity (natural of due to acquired immunization i.e. vaccine) of the permissive hosts force the virus in its natural cycle without apparent clinical manifestation in the hosts (e.g. Most by the arbovirus classically yellow fever, Dengue, Japanese encephalitis, West Nile, Zika etc.).

The *Paramyxoviridae* and *Rhabdoviridae* are the two other viral families in the order Mononegavirales, genetically closely related to the Filoviridae and having chiropteran as reservoir and/or vector [28]. Indeed, it is interesting to note that megachiropteran fruit bats are reservoirs of Hendra and Nipah viruses of the Paramyxoviridae family [29]. When, Microchiroptera bats are the probable ancestors of all rabies virus variants of the Lyssavirus genus in the family Rhabdoviridae and infecting presently terrestrial mammals [30]. Both also present this cryptic interepidemic silences that has not been yet clearly understood. The Nipah emerged one time in Malaysia (1999), thought to have its original cycle in PNG, and ultimately reemerged more than 3500 km away in Bangladesh in 2001. From its inception, again the Marburgvirus (the closest to EBOVs in the family of Filovirus), emerging events from an expected natural foci occurred within the path of time including 4 to 11 years of inter-epidemic silences occurring mostly in distant sites of Eastern and South Africa (Uganda, Zimbabwe, Angola, Kenya).

If one were to describe the history of Ebola outbreaks, one could simply construct a timeline, with a point on the line for each outbreak. You could create this timeline with a varying number of points, depending on your methodology, but regardless of how you built your timeline, there would be spaces between these points. This is due to the nature of Ebola; it appears, it disappears, and it appears again. To the Ebola virus, these gaps are periods of convalescence. To us, they are periods of absence and mystery, and one of these gaps stands out as the most mysterious (**Figure 1**).

The CDC lists five Ebola outbreaks in the late 1970's. The "first" Ebola outbreak took place in 1976, though we now recognize the event as two simultaneous and separate outbreaks. Between June and November 1976, 284 cases (151 deaths) of Ebola Sudan occurred near what is now Nzara, South Sudan; between September and October 1976, 318 cases (280 deaths) of Ebola Zaire occurred near what is now Yambuku, Democratic Republic of Congo (DRC). In November 1976, a researcher in England that was working with samples from the Nzara outbreak accidentally infected himself; CDC lists this accident as the third Ebola outbreak (the individual recovered). In June 1977, a child became sick and died from Ebola Zaire in Tandala, DRC though there was only one confirmed case, subsequent epidemiological investigations of the area uncovered several other historical, probable cases. Finally, between July and October 1979, 34 cases (22 deaths) of Ebola Sudan occurred, unbelievably, in Nzara, Sudan – the same community where the first cases of Ebola emerged just 3 years prior. In the span of just 39 months, the terror of Ebola had introduced itself to the world five times (638 cases, 454 deaths) and then... silence.

Ebola would not reappear for 10 whole years, and even then, the subtype was Ebola Reston, which we now know does not affect humans. Though CDC lists four Ebola Reston outbreaks between 1989 and 1992, the world would not see another case of Ebola virus disease in humans until late-1994, in Gabon. Even then, the outbreak (52 cases, 31 deaths) was mischaracterized as yellow fever for several months. Perhaps the virus's long absence from the spotlight had removed it from the collective consciousness in 1994, certainly in the presence of those pathogens that had been circulating and consuming our attention in the meantime.

This fifteen-year disappearance of Ebola, particularly in light of its frequent and severe outbreaks in the late 1970's, has perplexed researchers for decades.

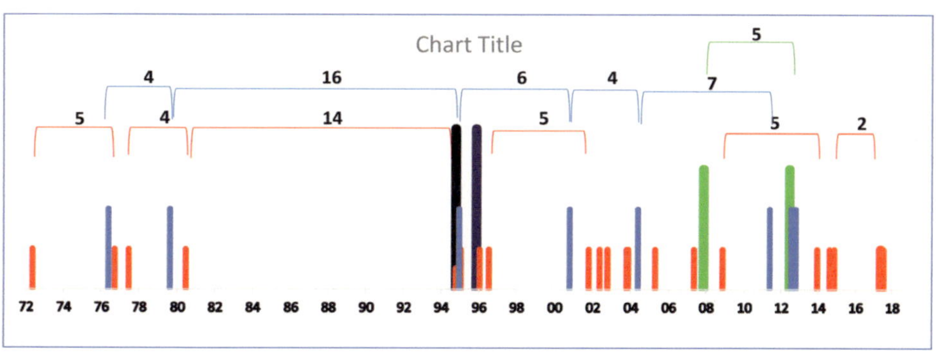

Figure 1.
Timeline of Ebolavirus emergence. Emerging events (bars) red = EBOV; blue = SEBOV; green = BDBV; horizontal axis = years 1972–2018; vertical axis = no value. Numbers above brackets = years of silent inter-emerging event.

The mystery lay, to some extent, within the lack of complete knowledge of the virus reservoir, though scientists are now having their long-held suspicions in bats confirmed. It's hard to detect disease when you cannot pinpoint the source. Surveillance and reporting have been another confounding element. How many times in that fifteen-year period was an illness misdiagnosed as yellow fever, dengue hemorrhagic fever, or some other similar illness, because of lack of knowledge or diagnostic capabilities, or simply because there was no health care around? We will probably never be able to answer this question. Finally, our perceived zone of endemicity at the time was limited to northern DRC and southern Sudan. Was the virus appearing elsewhere, unbeknownst to us? We certainly were not expecting it to emerge in Gabon in 1994, and Uganda in 2000, and West Africa in 2014 [31].

Scientists today continue to be perplexed by the emergence of the virus. What brings Ebola out from its hiding place? Is its emergence/re-emergence tied to climate change? globalization? the changing interface between humans and wildlife? If it has to do with any of these increasingly significant factors, how do they explain the fifteen-year disappearance?

These days, the virus comes and goes with some predictability—since 2000, outbreaks have approached a near-annual incidence, sometimes skipping a year, sometimes lasting more than a year. The periods between outbreaks are growing shorter. Is this because our capability to detect Ebola outbreaks is improving, or is the virus able to infect humans more frequently? One thing is for sure: the world knows that when one outbreak ends, another will eventually follow, and we need not wait 15 years.

4. Toward the discovery of the natural cycle of the Ebolaviruses

4.1 The discovery of a putative natural reservoir of Ebolavirus

Since the ZEBOV and SEBOV emergence, extended field studies have been conducted to discover the reservoir of EBOVs [32] including the 1976 first recorded DRC outbreaks and Sudan, the 1979 outbreak in DRC in 1979 and 1995 following the Kikwit outbreak, the same year in the Tai Forest and in 1999 in the Central African Republic [33–38] . A total of more than 7000 vertebrates and 30,000 invertebrates were sampled and tested for the presence of EBOVs. Limited finding was inconclusive for an potential EBOVs reservoir status among all these animals. Moreover, while several animal species (Bats, birds, reptiles, mollusks, arthropods, and plants) were experimentally infected with ZEBOV, only two fruit bat species (*Epomophorus* spp. and *Tadarida* spp.) developed a subclinical transient viremia [39]. If these results were not confirmed in the natural settings, they indicated the potential for chiropteran to be natural for EBOVs [40].

Also, historically, the first documented case of EVD in Sudan in 1976, the index case was located (by the World Health Organization) in a cotton factory far from the forest block, where the only wild significantly abundant species was an insectivorous bat species [21].

Since the discovery of EBOV in 1976, more than half of the epidemic outbreaks caused by EBOVs have broken down between Gabon and the DRC. Following the successive EBOV outbreaks in Gabon from 1995 to 2001 affecting several animal species non-human primates, and wild ungulates and responsible of the dramatic decline of great apes (gorilla and chimpanzee) populations in the region (Leroy et al. [16]), researchers engaged several missions of captures of wild animals in the forest areas affected by the recent past epidemics. Also, 1030 animals were captured and analyzed, only three species of fruit bats were found infected with the ZEBOV by PCR including: *Hypsignathus monstrosus*; *Epomops franqueti;* and *Myonycteris torquata*. Moreover, antibody reacting anti-Ebola were detected in these species as well as for the genus *Myonycteris* spp. leading ultimately to design Chiropteran as a potential reservoir of EBOVs [41].

Since then, many studies have converged in favor of the role of chiropters in maintaining EBOV in the wild (Caron et al. [42], Leendertz). In addition, a recent study of bats in Sierra Leone showed the association of an EBOV like with several species of bats (*Mops condylurus* and *Chaerephon pumilus*) from the Molossus family [43]. Moreover, a potential direct exposure to Ebola infected fruit bats was also reported as a putative index case of large epidemics [44, 45]. Moreover, further studies reported on direct infection of natural hosts (primates) by EBOV infected bats as highly plausible, given that bats, especially fruit bats, are frequently hunted and consumed as bushmeat by human when *Cercopithecus* species hunt roosting bats for consumption [46] also preying on bats has been reported in *Cercopithecus ascanius* and *C. mitis* (East Africa) as well as bonobos (DRC) [47]. It is also possible that different modes of exposure to Ebola virus could lead to different antibody profiles, that is, contaminated fruit vs. contact with infected bats during hunting [44, 47, 48].

Altogether, several fruit bats (*Epomophorus wahlbergi*) and insectivorous bats (*Chaerephon pumilus, Mops condylurus*) experimentally survive to EBOV infections [39], EBOV RNA and/or anti EBOV reacting antibodies were detected also in several other fruit bat species (*Epomops franqueti, Hypsignathus monstrosus, Myonycteris torquata*, *Eidolon helvum, Epomophorus gambianus, Micropteropus pusillus, Mops condylurus, Rousettus aegyptiacus, Rousettus leschenaultia*) giving more insight of the potential for chiropteran to be a potential host or reservoir host of EBOVs [22, 49, 50].

Interestingly, REBOV was also found associated with the bats in its natural habitat of the Philippines [51]. Also, again in this same *Filoviridae* family, Marburg viruses in Africa are clearly associated with bats [32, 52] as well as the Cueva virus in Europe [53]. While REBOV has been find associated with fruit bats, *Roussetus* spp. (Pteropodid family), each filovirus genus is associated with a specific chiropteran group including: Marburgvirus with a specific fruit bat, *Roussetus aegyptiacus* (Pteropodid family); and Cuevavirus with insectivorous bat, *Miniopterus schreibersii* (Miniopterid family); except for *Thamnovirus* isolated form fresh water fish.

Moreover, several virus groups are known to hold bat-borne viruses including the coronaviruses, hantaviruses, lyssaviruses, lassa virus, Henipavirus, filovirus which are among the most severe of the emerging viruses [54, 55].

Conclusively, this was the first evidence of chiropteran as a potential reservoir and/or vector of EBOV, while several wild animals, in particular great apes were find highly sensitive to EBOV infection. Also, if several species of chiropteran have been identified as a potential virus reservoir,

4.2 The most complete figure of a putative Ebolavirus natural cycle in the central African raining forest

From all above observations, records and historical events of EBOVs emerging events, several fundamentals of emergence have been identified as well putative time and space of such events where, that is when the virus jump from the cryptic natural cycle of the reservoir-vector to manifest itself clearly as an open index case of infection in a susceptible host and the potential opening epizootic or epidemic chain.

4.2.1 The actors

Again, from the literature numerous vertebrates appears to be permissive to infection by EBOVs, however, due to their ethology, including environmental habits, societal structure, density and their ability of intra and interspecies to mingle.

Altogether primates appear highly susceptible to EBOVs infection including non-human primate apes, gorilla and chimpanzee, but also cercopithecids (e.g. colobus) but also small wild ungulates (e.g. forest duikers) and eventually domestic animals (e.g. dogs) [32, 56–58].

One can summarize that EBOVs natural hosts belongs to chiropteran as a potential host reservoir represented mostly by Pteropodidae in Africa (REBOV and Roussetus; Bombali virus and Molossidae), and as secondary natural or accidental wild and domestic hosts including several other mammals: primates (Colobus, Cercopithecus), non-human primates (Gorilla, chimpanzee), wild ungulates (duikers) and, human primates. Also this needs to be taken into account with respect to other permissive species to EBOVs, indeed, as an example, if Roussetus spp. was shown to carry EBOVs reacting antibodies more recently *R. aegyptiacus* bats were demonstrated to unlikely able to maintain and perpetuate EBOV in nature while the natural transmission of filovirus in *R. aegyptiacus*, resulting viral replication and shedding are unknown [59].

4.2.2 The stages

The African Rain forest of the Congolese basin appears to be the epicenter of EBOVs emerging events. More than 80% of the emerging events of EBOVs occurred in the Tropical zone under the influence of the (Intertropical converging zone, ITCZ) from five degree North to 5 degrees south and oscillating as much as 40 to 45° of latitude north or south of the equator based on the pattern of land and ocean beneath it [28] (**Figure 2**).

Temperature and precipitation data for Africa (average data computed from 1960 to 1990, 300 m resolution [HIJ 05]) were integrated with the distribution map of the emergent events of the Ebola virus and the values calculated for each of the emergence points [60].

On all emergence points, the temperature at the time of emergence is not significantly different from the average annual temperature over 30 years. The difference in temperature between the moment of emergence and the average temperature (of 30 years monthly average) of the hottest month does not show any difference either. Emergence would not be directly related to temperature.

When we compare Ebolavirus emerging events time and the rainfall, there is strict quantitative correlation between rainfall and emergence: Most of the emergent events (93.8%) occurred during the rainy season (**Figure 2**). For precipitation values, there is a slightly statistically significant ($p = 0.02$) positive difference between the average precipitation of the month of emergence and the average of the monthly average precipitation (over 30 years), indicating that precipitations are higher when emergences occur. There is an even more statistically significant ($p = 0.003$) positive difference when considering precipitation of the month preceding the emergence. Emergence is therefore likely to be associated with rainfall intensity and the rainy season. 10/32 emergences occur at the beginning of the rainy season, 9/32 in the middle, and 11/32 at the end. Only 2/32 emergences occurred in the dry season.

When referring to land use (**Figure 3**) the temperature at the 6 emergence points in "Cropland" is highly significantly less ($p = 0.005$) than 15% (21.6°C) at temperature (24.4°C) to the 9 points in "Tree cover, broadleaved, evergreen, closed to open", however the average temperature of the Cropland (21.6°) is to a degree less, significantly lower ($p = 0.01$) than that of the "Tree cover" (24.5°C).

Ultimately, taking into account these environmental factors, when we look for an association between the emergent events of the Ebola virus and the

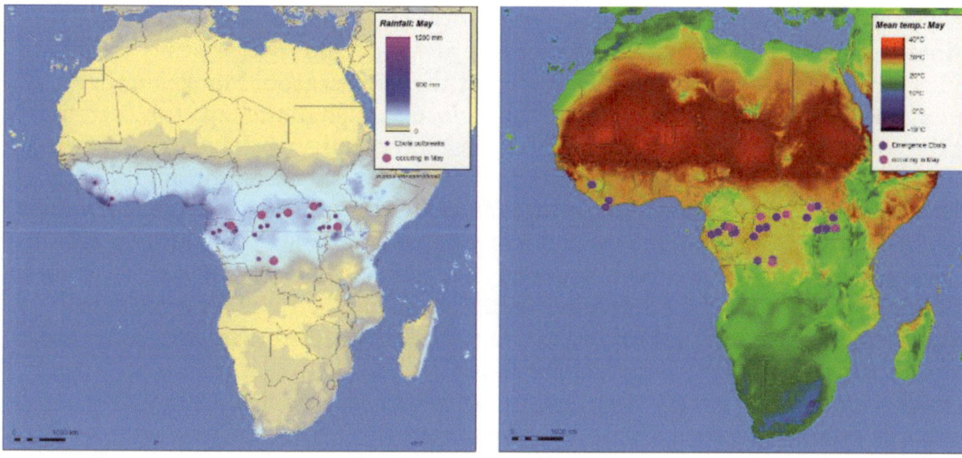

Figure 2.
Emerging events of Ebolavirus and climate since the Ebola fever inception in Africa. Left = annual rainfall; right = annual temperature. To illustrate the association temperature/rainfall and emergence, the month of May was chosen because it is at this time of the year that we observe the most emergent events of the Ebola virus. Temperature and rainfall are expressed as an annual average for the period under consideration. The precise location of 32 Ebola emergent events are here integrated into the global climatic map of Africa. Only 30-year average values per month of rainfall are available for the study period (ref.: WorldClim world databases) as well for the average monthly temperature.

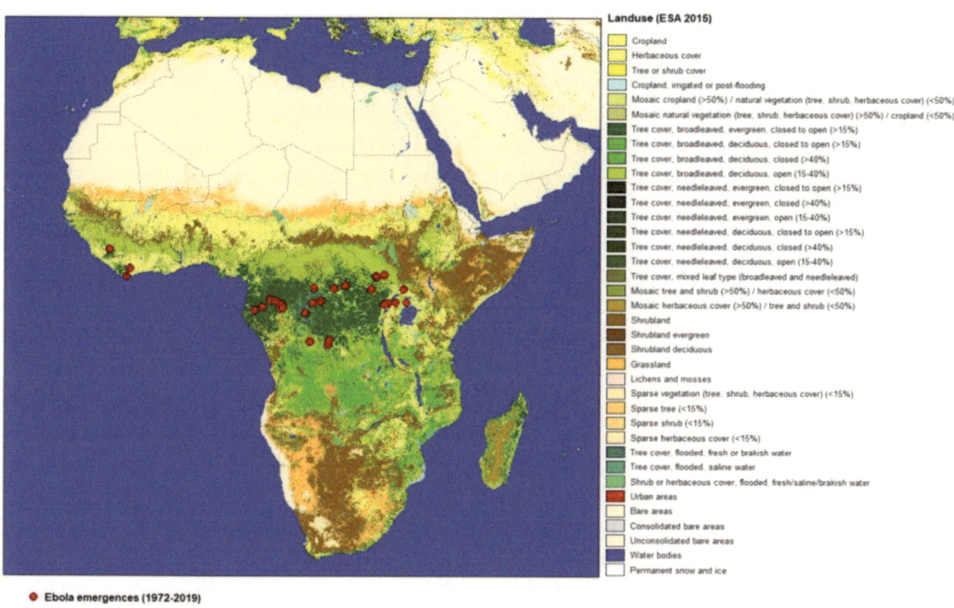

Figure 3.
Environmental factors surrounding Ebolavirus emerging event: Land use and places of Ebola virus emergence in Africa from 1976 to 2014. Land use from ESA 2015, 300 m resolution; red circle = putative place of the Ebola virus emergence (index case). Estimated Ebola emergence places are superimposed on the land use layer. The identification of the land use types were 32 points (red circle) representing the putative places of Ebolavirus emergence are superimposed and are distributed as follows: (1) cropland: 6, (2) herbaceous cover: 5, (3) cropland mosaic: 5 (> 50% natural vegetation vs. <50% tree, shrub, herbaceous cover), (4) tree cover with: (a) 15% of broadleaved, evergreen, closed to open: 9, (b) 15–40% of broadleaved, deciduous, open: 2, (5) flooded, fresh or brackish water: 1, (6) urban areas: 3, and (7) water bodies: 1. The limitations of this interpretation are linked to the accuracy of the location of Ebolavirus emergence sites (from literature and reports) and, to the evolution of vegetation cover over the past decades since the first emergence of the Ebolavirus occurred in Africa.

characteristics of the places of these emergences (i.e. land use, temperature, rainfall) it turns out that the emergences are always in the zone of heavy rainfall, but nevertheless do not follow the moving of the rainy season. Moreover, these emergences remain always and remarkably close enough to the Equator, therefore in the equatorial forest area with a high hygrometry, and a moderate annual temperature. However, the temperature at the time of emergence is not significantly different from the average annual temperature (at the points of emergence) which does not allow to distinguish seasonal effect in the emergence-temperature relationship. Conclusively, we did not identify a seasonality associated with the time of emergence, however the emerging events occur in specific geographic zone characterized by several environmental factors. Finally, the emergence zones are in areas of Land Use with specific temperatures not related to seasonality. Ultimately, it is also remarkable that all these emerging events occurred in an area with a highly potential presence of apes, virus-sensitive hosts.

4.2.3 Fundamentals and domains of emergence: a theory for a natural cycle of EBOVs in Africa

Also, the EBOVs species are closely genetically related, their seems to occur by foci in nature. The host appears to be the same, natural or accidental, and the transmission done by direct contact with infected hosts or its biological products [50, 61]. Altogether, in the early 2000s, before the identification of chiropteran as a potential host-reservoir of the EBOVs, a hypothetic natural cycle was described empirically based on seasonal environmental climatic factors [55]. Then, taking into account bats as a potential reservoir-host, the question of virus transmission was central to consider while environmental factors appears to play a major role to the host and their natural cycle (Chiropteran physiology) (climate/fructification, chorology, bats physiology). Several factors of emergence were then listed including: Chronic infection, infected organs, virus shedding, close encounters between reservoir and susceptible hosts, food and water resource, seasonality, chorology (i.e. causal effect between geographical phenomena – season) in the tropical rain forest and the spatial distribution of chiropteran (i.e. index site of Ebola emerging events).

Epidemiological field surveys indicate that mass mortalities of apes and monkey species due to Ebola virus often appear at the end of the dry season, a period when food resources are scarce. Restricted access to a limited number of fruit-bearing trees can lead to spatiotemporal clustering of diverse species of frugivorous animals, such as bats, nonhuman primates, and other terrestrial species foraging on fallen partially eaten (by bats) fruits. These aggregates of wild animal species favor the contact between infected and susceptible individuals and promote virus transmission. The dry season aggregation of reservoir host species involved in natural maintenance cycles, augmented by incidentally infected secondary hosts serving as sources for intra- and interspecific transmission chains independent of repeated spillover from the reservoir host, provides an ecological setting for amplifying enzootic transmission of Ebola virus when a vertebrate hosts are concentrated around a scarce number of water sources [62].

In addition to this dietary impoverishment, there are behavioral and physiological events occurring among bats during the tropical dry favor the contact frequency and intimacy between bats, which can promote transmission of Ebola virus to others and increase R0. As an example, megachiropteran fruit bats breeding activities and intraspecific competitions between males and grouped *kidding* of females favor the contact between individuals. Moreover, pregnancy can involve physiological changes among female bats that alter immune functions and eventually favor virus

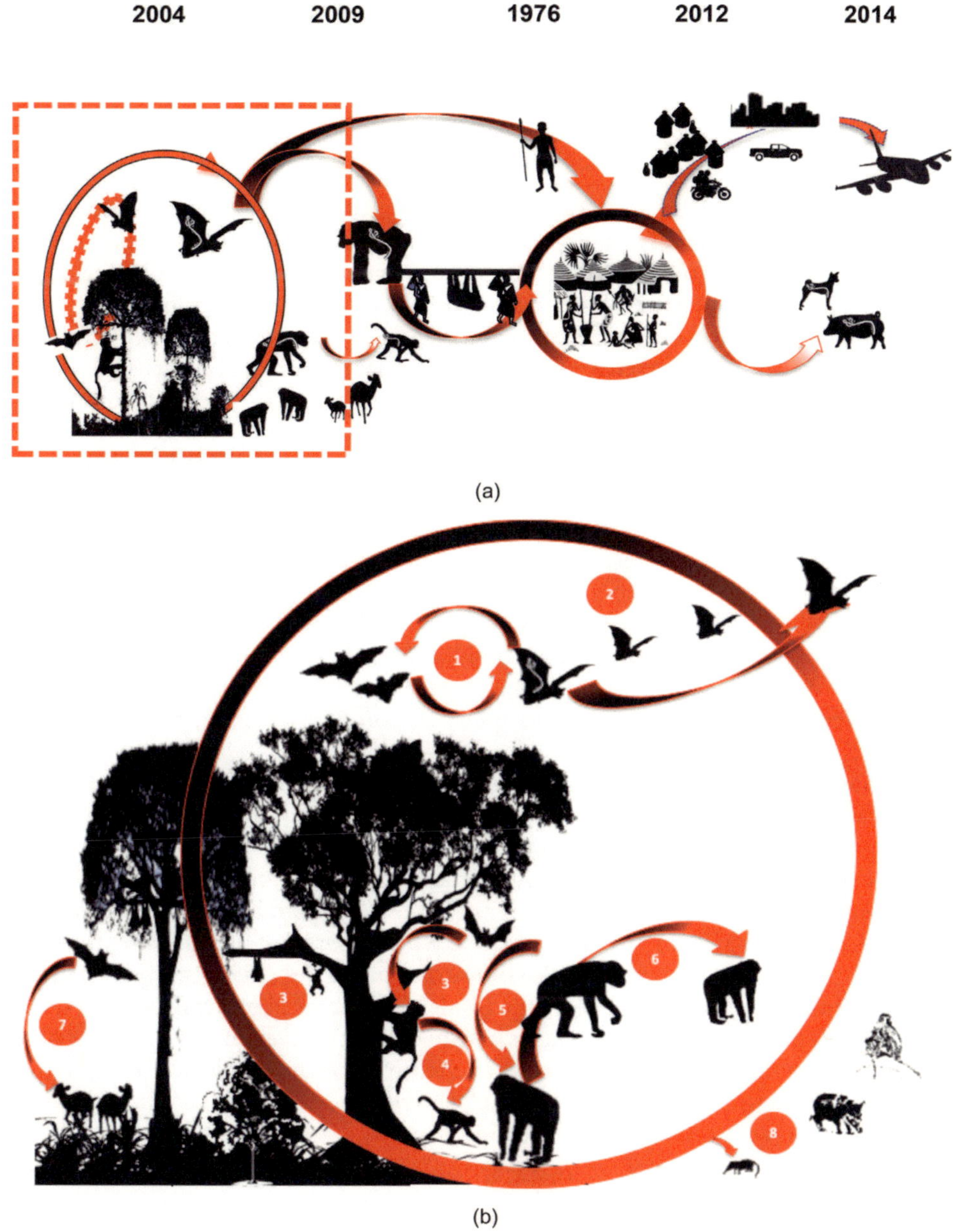

Figure 4.
(A) Understanding Ebolavirus enzootic and epidemics. Red arrows = cycles of transmission; dashed square = a putative natural cycle of Ebolavirus in Central Africa (see B). Fruit bats are considered to be a putative reservoir of Ebola virus in Central Africa after 2004; In 2009, several non-human primate epizootic are reported; 1976 was the first emerging events and subsequent epidemic chains in remote area of the rain forest and close by; 2012 showed a dramatic spread of the virus associated with motorized transportation and ground network; In 2014 urban epidemics are reported as well as a pandemic risk and become an international public health emergency. (B) Putative natural cycle of Ebolavirus in Central Africa. Red arrow indicates Ebolavirus transmission. Numbered red circle of transmission: (1) sylvatic inter- and intra-species transmission; (2) chiropteran migration; (3) chiropter to primate (close contact of dejection); (4) primate inter species (Cercopithecus/chimpanzee); (5) primate to primate (non-human primates); (6) non-human primate epizootic (gorillas); (7) chiropter to duikers; and (8) consumption of chiropteran infected food by shrew or wild pig.

shedding. Parturition among the African megachiropteran bats occurs throughout the year, although seasonal peaks provide birthing fluids, blood, and placental tissues, potentially Ebolavirus infected, falling on the ground as a medium highly attractive and readily available to scavenging terrestrial mammals [50, 56, 63] (**Figure 4A** and **B**).

5. If we had to conclude

Based on historical data and observations, the presented hypothesis of the natural cycle of Ebolavirus emergence prevail an inter-species spillover as the complex natural cycle involving several hosts (reservoir, vector, amplifier), as well as biotic and abiotic factors in a changing environment among other original features.

Although the natural cycle of EBOVs remains in the darkness of the rain forest, strong findings and comparative analysis of close parents of the filovirus throw some light to a potential natural cycle of EBOVs in Africa. EBOVs clearly appear linked to chiropteran and dependent for merging events in the environmental factors. Indeed, it appears that filoviridae are often associated with chiropteran while the emergence of the virus strains occurs as a sparse focus with a silent period of cryptic virus circulation. When virus transmission, i.e. spillover, from a hidden natural cycle, to accidental hosts occurs, it happened in a specific time-frame often linked to the season.

One can retain is that the EBOVs complex natural cycle is yet not on entirely elucidated and certainly dependent on environmental factors – associated with a specific environment of the chiropteran species incriminated (i.e. Different territories, different cycle) - leading to multiple, sometime concurrent, temporally and timely emergence in focus.

Although, other hypothesis has been suggested elsewhere including the Ebola virus Disease as an arthropod borne disease among others [42], there is important fundamental matters to consider as well before providing more.

However, beyond these hypotheses, fundamental questions subsist in order to go further learn. We can cite in particular the mystery of kin between the Reston virus of Asia and the Ebola viruses of Africa, would there not be a missing link in a geographic area yet to discover. Do the filovirus exist in the Americas hidden in the darkness of the tropical forest? Also, the Ebolavirus seems genetically stable, related to particular species of chiropter, was it to think about a co-evolution of the host and the virus in this closed environment of the forest of the tropical? Today, with the endless epidemic unfolding in the DRC, should we revisit our tools and strategy of struggle in an ever-changing world? [64].

Acknowledgements

We sincerely thank for their supports, brings to all the authors of this deep and never-ending research and scientific thought around an outstanding and fascinating subject: Georgetown University, Centaurus Biotech LLC., The DHS Emeritus Center for Emerging Zoonotic and Animal Diseases at Kansas State University.

Conflict of interest

All authors do not have any conflict of interest whatsoever with this published manuscript.

Author details

Jean-Paul Gonzalez[1,2*], Marc Souris[3], Massamba Sylla[4], Francisco Veas[2,5] and Tom Vincent[6]

1 Division of Biomedical Graduate Research Organization, Department of Microbiology and Immunology, School of Medicine, Georgetown University, Washington, DC, USA

2 Centaurus Biotech LLC, USA

3 Institute of Research for Development (IRD), Bondy, France

4 Ministry of Health, Senegal

5 Faculty of Pharmacy, Montpellier University, France

6 CRDF Global, USA

*Address all correspondence to: jpgonzalez2808@gmail.com

References

[1] CDC. Page last reviewed. Content source: Centers for Disease Control and Prevention, National Center for Emerging and Zoonotic Infectious Diseases (NCEZID), Division of High-Consequence Pathogens and Pathology (DHCPP), Viral Special Pathogens Branch (VSPB). 2019. Available from: https://www.cdc.gov/vhf/ebola/history/2014-2016-outbreak/index.html

[2] ICTV. Filoviridae. 2019. Available from: https://talk.ictvonline.org/ictv-reports/ictv_online_report/negative-sense-rna-viruses/mononegavirales/w/filoviridae

[3] Kuhn JH, Andersen KG, Baize S, Bào Y, Bavari S, Berthet N, et al. Nomenclature- and database-compatible names for the two Ebola virus variants that emerged in Guinea and the Democratic Republic of the Congo in 2014. Viruses. 2014;**6**(11):4760-4799. DOI: 10.3390/v6114760

[4] MacNeil A, Farnon EC, Morgan OW, et al. Filovirus outbreak detection and surveillance: Lessons from Bundibugyo. The Journal of Infectious Diseases. 2011;**204**:S761-S767

[5] Kiley MP, Bowen ET, Eddy GA, Isaäcson M, Johnson KM, McCormick JB, et al. Filoviridae: A taxonomic home for Marburg and Ebola viruses? Intervirology. 1982;**18**(1-2):24-32

[6] Anonymous. WHO/INTERNATIONAL STUDY TEAM. Ebola haemorrhagic fever in Zaire, 1976. Bulletin of the World Health Organization. 1978;**56**(2):271-293

[7] Anonymous. WHO/INTERNATIONAL STUDY TEAM. Ebola haemorrhagic fever in Sudan, 1976. Bulletin of the World Health Organization. 1978;**56**(2):247-270

[8] Centers for Disease Control. Ebola-Reston virus infection among quarantined nonhuman primates–Texas, 1996. Morbidity and Mortality Weekly Report. 1996;**45**:314-316

[9] Miranda MEG, Lee N, Miranda J. Reston ebolavirus in humans and animals in the Philippines: A review. The Journal of Infectious Diseases. 2011;**204**(suppl_3):S757-S760. DOI: 10.1093/infdis/jir296

[10] Le Guenno B, Formenty P, Wyers M, Gounon P, Walker F, Boesch C. Isolation and partial characterisation of a new strain of Ebola virus. The Lancet. 1995;**345**(8960):1271-1274

[11] Towner JS, Sealy TK, Khristova ML, Albariño CG, Conlan S, Reeder SA, et al. Newly discovered ebola virus associated with hemorrhagic fever outbreak in Uganda. PLoS Pathogens. 2008;**4**(11):e1000212. DOI: 10.1371/journal.ppat.1000212

[12] Miranda ME, Ksiazek TG, Retuya TJ, Khan AS, Sanchez A, Fulhorst CF, et al. Epidemiology of Ebola (subtype Reston) virus in the Philippines, 1996. The Journal of Infectious Diseases. 1999;**179**(Suppl 1):S115-S119

[13] Georges AJ, Leroy EM, Renaud AA, et al. Ebola hemorrhagic fever outbreaks in Gabon, 1994-1997: Epidemiologic and health control issues. The Journal of Infectious Diseases. 1999;**179**:S65-S75

[14] Baize S, Pannetier D, Oestereich L, Rieger T, Koivogui L, Magassouba N, et al. Emergence of Zaire Ebola virus disease in Guinea. The New England Journal of Medicine. 2014;**371**(15):1418-1425. DOI: 10.1056/NEJMoa1404505

[15] WHO. Disease Outbreak News. 2018a. Available from: https://www.who.int/ebola/situation-reports/drc-2018/en/ [Accessed: 13-01-19]

[16] Leroy EM, Rouquet P, Formenty P, Souquiere S, Kilbourne A, Froment JM, et al. Multiple Ebola virus transmission events and rapid decline of central African wildlife. Science. 2004a;**303**:387-390

[17] Heymann DL, Weisfeld JS, Webb PA, Johnson KM, Cairns T, Berquist H. Ebola hemorrhagic fever: Tandala, Zaire, 1977-1978. The Journal of Infectious Diseases. 1980;**142**:372-376

[18] O'Hearn AE, Voorhees MA, Fetterer DP, Wauquier N, Coomber MR, Bangura J, et al. Serosurveillance of viral pathogens circulating in West Africa. Virology Journal. 2016;**13**(1):163

[19] Becquart P, Wauquier N, Mahlakõiv T, Nkoghe D, Padilla C, Souris M, et al. High prevalence of both humoral and cellular immunity to *Zaire ebolavirus* among rural populations in Gabon. PLoS One. 2010;**5**(2):e9126

[20] Vincent T. Ebola Footprint—Broader Than You Think. Available from: http://oneill.law.georgetown.edu/the-ebola-footprint-broader-than-you-think/

[21] Olivero J, Fa JE, Real R, Farfan MA, Marquez AN, Vargas JM, et al. Mammalian biogeography and the Ebola virus in Africa. Mammal Review. 2016;**47**:24-37

[22] Olival KJ, Islam A, Yu M, Anthony SJ, Epstein JH, Khan SA, et al. Ebola virus antibodies in fruit bats, Bangladesh. Emerging Infectious Diseases. 2013;**19**:270-273. DOI: 10.3201/eid1902.120524

[23] Yuan JF, Zhang YJ, Li JL, Zhang YZ, Wang LF, Shi ZL. Serological evidence of ebolavirus infection in bats, China. Virology Journal. 2012;**9**:236. DOI: 10.1186/1743-422X-9-236

[24] Peterson AT, Bauer JT, Mills JN. Ecologic and geographic distribution of filovirus disease. Emerging Infectious Diseases. 2004;**10**:40-47. DOI: 10.3201/eid1001.030125

[25] Rollin PE, Williams RJ, Bressler DS, Pearson S, Cottingham M, Pucak G, et al. Ebola (subtype Reston) virus among quarantined nonhuman primates recently imported from the Philippines to the United States. The Journal of Infectious Diseases. 1999;**179**(Suppl 1):S108-S114

[26] Wauquier N, Bangura J, Moses L, Humarr Khan S, Coomber M, Lungay V, et al. Understanding the emergence of ebola virus disease in Sierra Leone: Stalking the virus in the threatening wake of emergence. PLOS Currents. 2015;7

[27] Ebola virus cases in the United States. Available from: https://en.wikipedia.org/wiki/Ebola_virus_cases_in_the_United_States

[28] Monath TP. Ecology of Marburg and Ebola viruses: Speculations and directions for the future research. The Journal of Infectious Diseases. 1999;**179**:S127-S138

[29] Yob JM, Field H, Rashdi AM, Morrissy C, van der Heide B, Rota P, et al. Nipah virus infection in bats (order Chiroptera) in peninsular Malaysia. Emerging Infectious Diseases. 2001;**7**(3):439-441

[30] Badrane H, Tordo N. Host switching in Lyssavirus history from the Chiroptera to the Carnivora orders. Journal of Virology. 2001;**75**:8096-8104

[31] Tom Vincent. EBOLA: FIFTEEN YEARS OF SILENCE. 2019. Available from: http://oneill.law.georgetown.edu/ebola-fifteen-years-of-silence/

[32] Pourrut X, Souris M, Towner JS, Rollin PE, Nichol ST, Gonzalez JP,

et al. Large serological survey showing cocirculation of Ebola and Marburg viruses in Gabonese bat populations, and a high seroprevalence of both viruses in Rousettus aegyptiacus. BMC Infectious Diseases. 2009;**9**:159

[33] Breman JG, Johnson KM, van der Groen G, Robbins CB, Szczeniowski MV, Ruti K, et al. A search for Ebola virus in animals in the Democratic Republic of the Congo and Cameroon: Ecologic, virologic, and sero- logic surveys, 1979-1980. The Journal of Infectious Diseases. 1999;**179**:S139-S147

[34] Arata AA, Johnson B. Approaches towards studies on potential reservoirs of viral haemorrhagic fever in southern Sudan. In: Pattyn SR, editor. Ebola Virus Haemor- Rhagic Fever. Amsterdam: Elsevier/Netherland biomedical; 1977. pp. 191-202

[35] Leirs H, Mills JN, Krebs JW, Childs JE, Akaibe D, Woollen N, et al. Search for the Ebola virus reservoir in Kikwit Democratic Republic of the Congo: Reflections on a vertebrate collection. The Journal of Infectious Diseases. 1999;**179**:S155-S163

[36] Morvan JM, Deubel V, Gounon P, Nakoune E, Barriere P, Murri S, et al. Identification of Ebola virus sequences present as RNA or DNA in organs of terrestrial small mammals of the Central African Republic. Microbes and Infection. 1999;**1**:1193-1201

[37] Reiter P, Turell M, Coleman R, Miller B, Maupin G, Liz J, et al. Field investigations of an outbreak of Ebola hemorrhagic fever Kikwit Democratic Republic of the Congo, 1995: Arthropod studies. The Journal of Infectious Diseases. 1999;**179**:S148-S154

[38] Formenty P, Boesch C, Wyers M, Steiner C, Donati F, Dind F, Walker F, Le Guenno B. Ebola virus outbreak among wild chimpanzees living in a rain forest of cote d'Ivoire. The Journal of Infectious Diseases. 1999;**179**(Suppl 1): S120-S126

[39] Swanepoel R, Leman PA, Burt FJ. Experimental inoculation of plants and animals with Ebola virus. Emerging Infectious Diseases. 1996;**2**:321-325

[40] Xavier P, Gonzalez JP, Leroy E. Spatial and temporal patterns of Ebola virus antibody prevalence in the putative bat species reservoir. The Journal of Infectious Diseases. 2007;**196**(Suppl 2):S176-S183

[41] Eric L, Kumulungui B, Pourrut X, Rouquet P, Yaba P, Délicat A, et al. Fruit bats as reservoirs of Ebola virus. Nature. 2005;**438**(7068):575-576

[42] Caron A, Bourgarel M, Cappelle J, Liégeois F, De Nys HM, Roger F. Ebola virus maintenance: If not (only) bats, what Else? Viruses. 2018;**10**(10):549. DOI: 10.3390/v10100549

[43] Goldstein T, Anthony SJ, Gbakima A, Bird BH, Bangura J, Tremeau-Bravard A, et al. The discovery of Bombali virus adds further support for bats as hosts of ebolaviruses. Nature Microbiology. 2018;**3**:1084-1089

[44] Leroy EM, Epelboin A, Mondonge V, Pourrut X, Gonzalez JP, Muyembe-Tamfum JJ, et al. Ebola outbreak associated with direct exposure to fruit bats in Luebo, Democratic Republic of the Congo, 2007. Vector Borne and Zoonotic Diseases. 2009;**9**(6):723-728

[45] Marí Saéz A, Weiss S, Nowak K, Lapeyre V, Zimmermann F, Düx A, et al. Investigating the zoonotic origin of the west African Ebola epidemic. EMBO Molecular Medicine. 2015;7(1):17-23. DOI: 10.15252/emmm.201404792

[46] Tapanes E, Detwiler KM, Cords M. Bat predation by Cercopithecus monkeys: Implications for zoonotic disease transmission. EcoHealth. 2016;**13**:405-409

[47] Bermejo M, Illera G, Sabater P. Animals and mushrooms consumed by bonobos (pan paniscus): New records from Lilungu (Ikele), Zaire. International Journal of Primatology. 1994;**15**:879-898

[48] Leendertz SAJ, Gogarten JF, Düx A, Calvignac-Spencer S, Leendertz FH. Assessing the evidence supporting fruit bats as the primary reservoirs for Ebola viruses. EcoHealth. 2016;**13**(1):18-25

[49] Olival KJ, Hayman DT. Filoviruses in bats: Current knowledge and future directions. Viruses. 2014;**6**(4):1759-1788. DOI: 10.3390/v6041759

[50] Gonzalez JP, Pourrut X, Leroy E. Ebolavirus and other filoviruses. Current Topics in Microbiology and Immunology. 2007;**315**:363-387

[51] Jayme SI, Field HE, de Jong C, Olival KJ, Marsh G, Tagtag AM, et al. Molecular evidence of Ebola Reston virus infection in Philippine bats. Virology Journal. 2015;**12**:107. DOI: 10.1186/s12985-015-0331-3

[52] Pawęska JT, Jansen van Vuren P, Kemp A, Storm N, Grobbelaar AA, Wiley MR, et al. Marburg virus infection in Egyptian Rousette bats, South Africa, 2013-20141. Emerging Infectious Diseases. 2018 Jun;**24**(6):1134-1137. DOI: 10.3201/eid2406.172165

[53] de Arellano ER, Sanchez-Lockhart M, Perteguer MJ, Bartlett M, Ortiz M, Campioli P, et al. First evidence of antibodies against Lloviu virus in Schreiber's bent-winged insectivorous bats demonstrate a wide circulation of the virus in Spain. Viruses. 2019;**11**:360. DOI: 10.3390/v11040360

[54] Calisher CH, Childs JE, Field HE, Holmes KV, Schountz T. Bats: Important reservoir hosts of emerging viruses. Clinical Microbiology Reviews. 2006;**19**:531-545

[55] Gonzalez JP, Pourrut X, Leroy E. Ebolavirus and other filoviruses. In: Childs JE, Mackenzie JS, Richt JA, editors. Wildlife and Emerging Zoonotic Diseases: The Biology, Circumstances and Consequences of Cross-Species Transmission. New York, NY, USA: Springer; Heidelberg, Germany; 2007. pp. 363-388

[56] Allela L, Bourry O, Pouillot R, Délicat A, Yaba P, Kumulungui B, et al. Ebola virus antibody in dogs and human risk. Emerging Infectious Diseases. 2005;**11**(3):385-390

[57] Ayouba A, Ahuka-Mundeke S, Butel C, Mbala Kingebeni P, Loul S, Tagg N, et al. Extensive serological survey of multiple African non-human primate species reveals low prevalence of IgG antibodies to four Ebola virus species. The Journal of Infectious Diseases. 2019. DOI: 10.1093/infdis/jiz006

[58] Pigott DM, Golding N, Mylne A, et al. Mapping the zoonotic niche of Ebola virus disease in Africa. eLife. 2014;**3**:e04395

[59] Paweska JT, Storm N, Grobbelaar AA, Markotter W, Kemp A, Jansen van Vuren P. Experimental inoculation of Egyptian fruit bats (*Rousettus aegyptiacus*) with Ebola virus. Viruses. 2016;**8**(2). pii: E29. DOI: 10.3390/v8020029

[60] Hijmans RJ, Cameron SE, Parra JL, Jones PG, Jarvis A. Very high-resolution interpolated climate surfaces for global land areas. International Journal of Climatology. 2005;**25**:1965-1978

[61] Mackensie J, Mills J, editors. Review. In: Wildlife and Emerging Zoonotic Diseases. Springer-Verelag CRC Press. Advances in Virology ch20

[62] Shaman J, Day JF, Stieglitz M. Drought-induced amplification of Saint Louis encephalitis virus Florida. Emerging Infectious Diseases. 2002;**8**:575-580

[63] Pourrut X, Kumulungui B, Wittmann T, Moussavou G, Delicat A, Yaba P, et al. The natural history of Ebola virus in Africa. Microbes and Infection. 2005;**7**(7-8):1005-1014

[64] Gonzalez JP, Souris M, Valdivia-Granda W. Global spread of hemorrhagic fever viruses: Predicting pandemics. Methods in Molecular Biology. 2018;**1604**:3-31. DOI: 10.1007/978-1-4939-6981-4_1

Section 3

Clinical Features

Chapter 3

Maternal Filovirus Infection and Death from Marburg and Ravn Viruses: Highly Lethal to Pregnant Women and Their Fetuses Similar to Ebola Virus

David A. Schwartz

Abstract

Ebola virus and the marburgviruses are distinct filoviruses that share common clinical presentations and clinical management protocols. However, the marburgviruses are not as well known as is their close relative, Ebola virus, and are a much less frequent cause of human outbreaks. Marburg virus disease (MVD) is caused by two marburgviruses that are clinically indistinguishable—Marburg virus and Ravn virus. There is scant information available concerning MVD in pregnancy, but it appears clear that, similar to Ebola virus, MVD infection is associated with an extremely high maternal and fetal mortality rate. This chapter will examine what is known about Marburg and Ravn virus infections in pregnant women, their clinical outcomes, and the pathogenesis of MVD in experimental animal models of infection. These data will be compared with the more comprehensive information available regarding Ebola virus disease in pregnancy including its effects on pregnant women and the fetus.

Keywords: Ebola virus, Marburg virus, Ravn virus, pregnancy, maternal death, fetal death, filovirus, maternal infection, hemorrhagic fever, maternal mortality, maternal morbidity, fetal mortality, West African Ebola epidemic, epidemiology

1. Introduction

The Ebola and Marburg viruses are distinct filoviruses that share common clinical presentations and clinical management protocols. However, the Marburg virus is not as well-known as its relative, the Ebola virus. The largest Ebola epidemic in history occurred in West Africa from 2013 to 2015 in which 28,616 persons were reported to be infected. Following a small outbreak of 54 probable and confirmed cases in the Équateur Province of the Democratic Republic of the Congo (DRC) from May to June 2018, a second and larger epidemic has occurred in the Kivu and North Ituri Provinces since August 2018 [1]. This epidemic has infected 2592 persons as of July 2019 and is the second largest Ebola epidemic in history. In contrast to the Ebola virus, Marburg virus disease (MVD) occurs much less frequently. MVD is caused by two marburgviruses that are clinically indistinguishable—the Marburg

IntechOpen

virus (MARV) and Ravn virus (RAVV). Including occurrences of MVD in less than 5 persons, there have been 13 outbreaks of MVD, with the largest reported from DRC between 1998 and 2000 (154 persons infected) and in Angola between 2004 and 2005 (252 persons infected) [2]. As can be seen, the scale of MVD outbreaks has been much less than those of its filovirus relative Ebola virus.

2. The marburgviruses

The marburgviruses are single-stranded RNA viruses belonging to the family *Filoviridae*, which also includes the *Ebolavirus* genus. The genus *Marburgvirus* comprises a single species, *Marburg marburgvirus*, that includes two variants - the Marburg virus (MARV) and the Ravn virus (RAVV) [3, 4]. Similar to other members of the family *Filoviridae*, marburgvirions have a filamentous configuration that appears by electron microscopy to resemble a shepherd's crook, or in the shape of a "U" or a "6"; coiled, toroid, or branched forms can be seen (**Figure 1**). The marburgviruses cause a severe viral illness in humans termed Marburg virus disease, or MVD (formerly termed Marburg hemorrhagic fever). Illness due to the marburgviruses is clinically indistinguishable from Ebola virus disease (EVD). Although Marburg virus disease and Ebola virus disease have historically been labeled as hemorrhagic fevers, hemorrhage is found in less than 50% of patients [5]. According to some authors, they may be considered as gastrointestinal diseases that develop severe systemic organ involvement including hemorrhages [6]. After an incubation period that varies between 4 and 10 days, infected individuals abruptly develop flu-like symptoms characterized by fever, chills, malaise, and myalgia. This is followed by signs and symptoms indicating systemic involvement, including prostration and gastrointestinal symptoms (anorexia, nausea, vomiting, abdominal pain, and diarrhea), respiratory complaints (chest pain, shortness of breath, and cough), vascular findings (conjunctival injection, postural hypotension, and edema), and neurological symptoms (headache, confusion, and coma). The typical hemorrhagic manifestations of

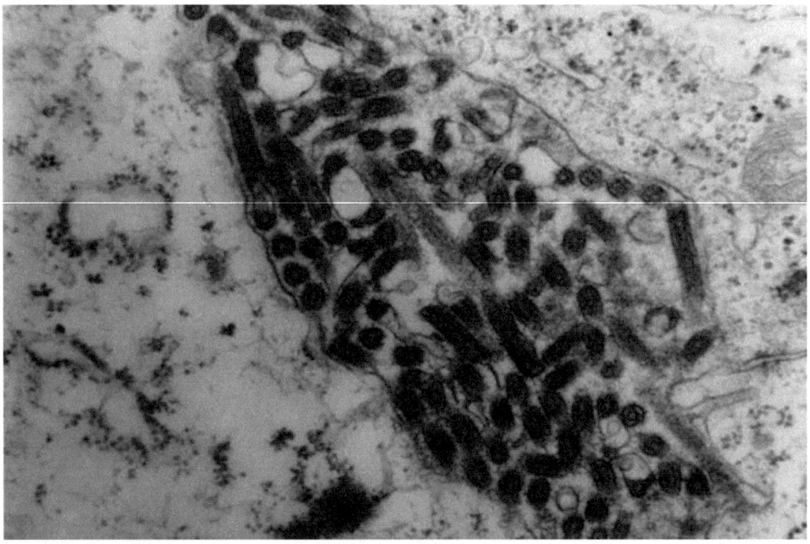

Figure 1.
Transmission electron micrograph demonstrating the typical filovirus morphology of Marburg virus. This specimen was obtained from an infected person who acquired the infection in 1975 while traveling through Rhodesia (now Zimbabwe). Photograph courtesy of the US Centers for Disease Control and Prevention, Atlanta, USA.

MVD include purpura, ecchymoses, petechiae, maculopapular rash, and hematomas, with death rapidly ensuing as a result of multiple organ dysfunction syndrome (MODS) and disseminated intravascular coagulation (DIC), hypotension, fluid redistribution, and focal tissue necrosis. MVD (and EVD) can be confused with other infectious diseases occurring in Equatorial Africa including other hemorrhagic fevers, falciparum malaria, rickettsial diseases, typhoid fever, and more.

3. Epidemiology of Marburg virus disease

The majority of cases of primary MVD acquired in Africa have been associated with persons visiting caves or working in mines, locations where bats are common. Egyptian fruit bats (rousette bats, *Rousettus aegyptiacus*) (**Figure 2**) have been found to represent a major natural reservoir and source of marburgviruses [7]; the bats do not develop illness from the virus. Infected Egyptian rousette bats may shed marburgviruses in their saliva, urine, and feces as they feed on fruit which can then be transmitted to humans. Direct contact with infected bats can also transmit the virus, such as through bites. In December 2018 it was disclosed that five Egyptian rousette bats tested positive for Marburg virus in Sierra Leone—the first time that the virus was identified in West Africa [8]. Two of the four strains identified among the five Marburg-positive bats in Sierra Leone have genetic similarity to the strain of MARV that caused the MVD outbreak in Angola. This was the first time scientists detected these Angolan strains in bats [9]. Another risk factor for acquiring MVD is physical contact with nonhuman primates, although there has been just one outbreak of MVD, in 1967, that resulted from contact with infected monkeys. Transmission of the virus can also occur by handling ill or dead infected wild animals. Mathematical models of the potential geographic distribution of the marburgviruses have indicated that the potential range of the virus includes a broad distribution across the arid woodlands of Equatorial Africa, with possible distribution through eastern and southern Africa as well [10].

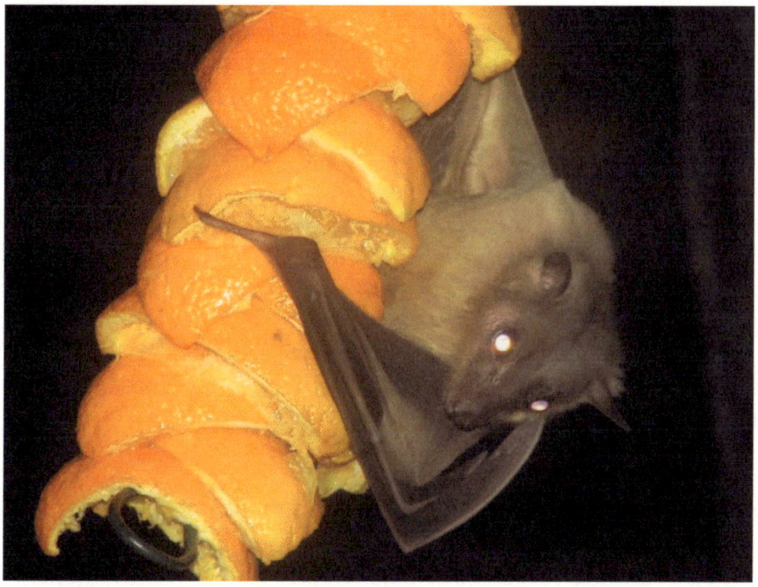

Figure 2.
An Egyptian fruit bat (Rousettus aegyptiacus) clings to pieces of orange at the Cotswold Wildlife Park, England. Photograph from Adrian Pingstone and Wikipedia.

The marburgviruses are transmitted from person-to-person through direct and unprotected contact with blood, body fluids, and tissues of infected persons. Risk factors for acquiring secondary MVD include close contact with severely ill patients or their body fluids in the acute phase of the disease, either at home or in a hospital, thus placing caregivers at risk for acquiring the infection. In addition, unsafe burial practices are common routes of infection. These are the identical mechanisms for transmission for Ebola virus. MVD has not been reported to be transmitted via the aerosol route. Women who are pregnant and infected with either marburgviruses or Ebola virus can be especially infectious—the placenta has a high viral load, and maternal blood, vaginal secretions, amniotic fluid, urine, sweat, saliva, feces, vomit, and breast milk are all potential sources of virus [11]. Products of conception as occur in miscarriages can also be infectious, as can fetal tissues.

Based upon the history of primary MVD infection occurring in association with exposure to bat-infested caves and mines and additional environmental and occupational risk factors for acquiring the infection, it appears unlikely that Marburg virus infection of a pregnant woman would occur as the index case of an outbreak. Thus, unlike the situation of some viral infections (notably hepatitis E) where infections in pregnant women can represent the index cases of a community-wide outbreak [12], MVD occurring in pregnant women would likely represent secondary infections within the community, prompting an epidemiological investigation to identify the index case(s). During the West Africa Ebola epidemic, pregnant women often became infected through the traditional female roles of caregiver to the sick as well as through preparation of the dead and via unsafe burials [13]. The high rate of transmissibility of filoviral infections was demonstrated in one Liberian village named Joe Blow Town. There, all of the mothers in the town became infected and died after acquiring EVD after caring for a woman who was infected and, following her death, preparing her body and then bathing in the water that had been used to wash her corpse [14].

Following acute infection, both marburgviruses and Ebola virus can persist in a variety of bodily fluids. Ebola virus and Marburg virus have both been found by culture from ocular aqueous humor 2 and 3 months after disease onset, respectively. Ebola virus RNA has been identified in breast milk for up to 21 days after the onset of the disease and in vaginal secretions up to 33 days after its onset. In one report, a 9-month-old infant is believed to have acquired Ebola virus infection through breastfeeding from a mother who did not report having a febrile illness—persistent Ebola virus RNA was identified in both the mother's breast milk and in the father's seminal fluid [15].

In men, Ebola virus has been identified in the semen of survivors for many months after acute infection, with some having persistence of Ebola RNA for up to 18 months [16]. It is likely that the marburgviruses would also demonstrate persistence in seminal fluid of male survivors. Sexual transmission of marburgviruses was reported in 1968 after the initial outbreak of Marburg virus disease [17]. In a study in crab-eating macaques, it was found by Coffin et al. [18] that experimentally infected males had persistent MARV infection of the seminiferous tubules, an immunologically privileged site. Affecting primarily the Sertoli cells, this viral persistence resulted in severe testicular damage including spermatogenic cell depletion, inflammation, and breakdown of the blood-testis barrier [18].

4. Outbreaks of Marburg virus disease

Marburg virus disease was initially discovered in 1967 when 31 persons unexplainably became ill in the cities of Marburg and Frankfurt am Main in Germany and Belgrade in the former Yugoslavia. The illness was traced to exposure to tissues or cell cultures obtained from a group of imported African green monkeys (grivets or *Chlorocebus aethiops*) that were originally from Uganda and had been maintained for making antisera in commercial laboratories. All the patients in Marburg were employees of Behringwerke, which produced sera and vaccines, and the infected persons in Frankfurt were employees of the Paul Ehrlich Institute, a control institute for sera and vaccines. All of the persons who developed a primary infection at the three locations had direct contact with blood, organs, and cell cultures from *Cercopithecus aethiops* monkeys. This initial outbreak resulted in 25 primary MARV infections including 7 deaths and 6 nonfatal secondary cases occurring in the persons and who treated them and their family members [19, 20].

Since this initial recognition of the virus in Europe, there have been at least 12 additional episodes or outbreaks of MVD in humans (**Figure 3**). Numbers of infected individuals have varied, some episodes having only one person involved,

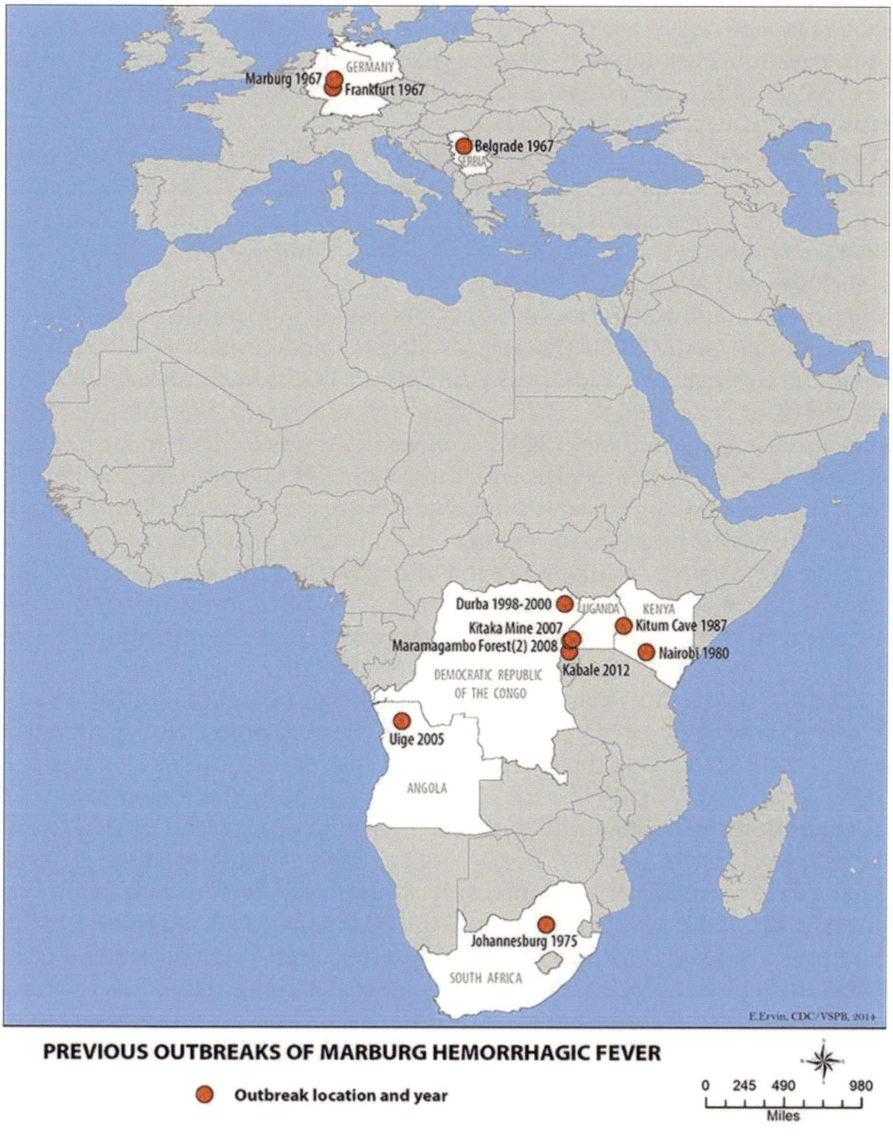

Figure 3.
Distribution of outbreaks of Marburg virus disease from 1967 to 2012. The 2014 infection of a single individual in Uganda and the 2017 outbreak in Kween, Uganda, are not indicated on this map. Photograph from the US Centers for Disease Control and Prevention, Atlanta, USA.

others involving an infected individual and a care provider, while in one outbreak as many as 252 persons were infected.

In February of 1975, the first outbreak of MVD to occur in Africa was recognized in a young Australian man who acquired the infection while traveling in Rhodesia (now Zimbabwe). He died in a Johannesburg hospital on the 7th day of infection. Two secondary cases developed—a traveling companion and a nurse—and both survived [21].

In 1980 a French electrical engineer working in Nzoia, Kenya, in a sugar factory acquired MVD and died shortly after admission to Nairobi Hospital. His attending physician also contracted MVD but survived [22]. Although it remains unknown how he acquired his infection, he worked at the base of Mount Elgon, where Kitum Cave is located. Kitum cave, 165 meters long and up to 60 meters wide with walls rich in salt, is inhabited by thousands of Egyptian fruit bats as well as by other bat species.

A 15-year-old boy from Denmark developed MVD infection during a visit to Kenya in 1987. He had visited a cave—Kitum Cave—on Mount Elgon and subsequently traveled to Mombasa where he was noted to be ill. He died following transfer to Nairobi Hospital [23]. The causative agent was later found to be a new strain of MVD—the Ravn virus—and thus this was first report of this marburgvirus agent and its causes with human disease.

Two laboratory-acquired infections occurred with MARV occurred in the former Soviet Union in 1988 and 1990. Scant information is available regarding these events, although in one case it is known that the individual became infected after an accidental self-inoculation of MARV with a syringe while working with guinea pigs and which resulted in his death [24, 25].

A major epidemic of MVD occurred in 1998 among gold miners from the Goroumbwa mine in the DRC. This was the largest epidemic to have occurred up to that time and continued sporadically in the cities of Durba and Watsa up to 2000. A total of 154 cases occurred (48 confirmed and 106 suspected), with 52% in young male miners. The large majority (94%) of infected miners worked underground, and cessation of the outbreak coincided with the flooding of the mine [26]. Retrospective virologic and epidemiologic analysis revealed evidence for multiple introductions of MARV and RAVV viruses into the population as there were at least nine genetically distinct lineages of virus circulating during the outbreak [26]. This epidemic had a case fatality rate of 83% and importantly was the first MVD outbreak to report infection of pregnant women and their infants (see below). It also significantly affected children and early teens—for the 145 patients for whom demographic data were available, 18 of them (12%) were under the age of 15 years including 15 infants [26].

The largest outbreak of MVD to develop in Africa began in October 2004 in Angola [27, 28]. Centered in the northeastern Uige Province, this epidemic was not identified as being due to MVD until March 2005 following the transmission of the disease to healthcare workers, which alerted the community to the possibility of Marburg or Ebola virus disease. The outbreak persisted until July 2005 [29], and eventually there were 252 persons infected, of whom 227 died—a case fatality rate of approximately 90% [29, 30]. Case finding and follow-up during this outbreak was hampered by several factors. Individuals and patients often resisted medical assistance and epidemiologic studies because of circulating rumors that the foreign teams were responsible for bringing or spreading the virus. Clandestine practices including families hiding ill members, avoiding going to the hospital, immediately burying the deceased, utilizing native healers, and bringing patients to hospitals just before death suggest that the true severity of the outbreak and data on morbidity and lethality might never be known. In addition, patient records were maintained only upon admission and not during hospitalization [31]. Approximately 75% of the reported cases had occurred in children aged 5 years or younger [32]. There were no available data on the number of pregnant women, if any, who became infected during this large outbreak. However, a report from Jeffs et al. and Médecins Sans Frontières (MSF) [33] working at the Uige Provincial Hospital, the initial epicenter of the outbreak, confirmed that screening for MVD was performed in the maternity ward of the hospital. Assessment of pregnant women was particularly challenging, and many of these women were febrile and fulfilled the suspected case definition for MVD, especially as bleeding during pregnancy is common. The authors [33] stated:

> *"It was often difficult to rule out MHF without testing, but, because many women required constant obstetric assistance, it would have been difficult to admit them all to the formal Marburg ward for assessment. Therefore, a well-equipped isolation area was set up in the maternity ward, including a delivery area and a ward area. Maternity staff were trained in infection control, and separate teams were assigned to the isolation area and the normal maternity ward. Any patient testing positive for MHF was admitted to the Marburg ward."*

Thus, it would appear that there were possible cases of pregnant women with infection during the Uige outbreak, but that cannot be confirmed.

Between 2007 and 2008, there were two outbreaks of MVD in Southwest Uganda—one among miners working in Kitaka Mine in the Kamwenge District [34] and the other in two tourists, one Dutch and the other American, that had separately visited Python Cave in Queen Elizabeth National Park [35, 36]. Both Python Cave and the Kitaka mine are inhabited by Egyptian fruit bats (*Rousettus aegyptiacus*) [37].

An outbreak of MVD was declared in October 2012 in the western Uganda districts of Kabale, Ibanda, and Kamwenge [38] that resulted in 20 confirmed or probable cases and 9 deaths. This outbreak was also linked to mining activity in the Ibanda District.

In September 2014 a 30-year-old male healthcare worker (radiographer) developed symptoms of a viral hemorrhagic fever. Following 1 week of illness, he was admitted to a district health facility in the Mpigi District and later transferred to a hospital in Kampala, Uganda. He expired 2 weeks after the onset of illness, and it was later confirmed that he was infected with MARV. The source of his infection was not identified, and there were no other infected persons identified [37, 39].

In October 2017 an outbreak of MVD occurred in the Kween District of Uganda, near the border with Kenya [40, 41]. The initial three infected persons all belonged to the same family and died. The (probable) initially infected person was a 35-year-old herdsman who frequently hunted near the area of Kaptum, which is known for its bat-infested caves. A healthcare worker also became infected.

5. Marburg virus disease in pregnant women, fetuses, and infants

There is very little information available on the effects of MVD on pregnant women, their fetuses, and infants, including clinical obstetrical and neonatal outcomes following MVD infection and the persistence of virus post-infection. Similar to some of the initial outbreaks of Ebola virus disease, the pregnancy status of women suspected or confirmed as having MVD was not generally recorded during outbreaks and may not have even been evaluated at the time of their illness [1].

Based upon the reported cases of filovirus infections occurring in pregnancy, there is no evidence that women who are pregnant are more susceptible to becoming infected with either marburgviruses or the Ebola virus [6]. However, it does appear that once they acquire a filovirus infection, pregnant women are more likely to have a fatal outcome than are nonpregnant individuals [1, 6]. Pregnant women with EVD and MVD are at high risk of spontaneous abortion and stillbirth. EVD is associated with pregnancy-related hemorrhage, and although it has not been reported, it can probably also complicate MVD infection. Evidence from a number of reports confirms that hematogenous spread of *Filovirus* infection through the placenta is the most common source of fetal infection, as high viral titers have been detected in placental tissue not only for Ebola but also for other hemorrhagic fever viruses [11].

The initial report of MVD occurring in pregnant women and fetuses was derived from the outbreak occurring in the gold mining village of Dursa and district capital of Watsa in the DR Congo in 1998–1999 [6, 26]. During this outbreak, at least three pregnant women with MVD were reported, all of whom died. The infection was also lethal for their infants—one woman had a miscarriage, and another delivered an infant who died 7 h after birth. Thus, the only information available on the clinical effects of MVD occurring in pregnant women indicates a 100% case fatality rate among infected mothers and their infants. This is higher than the mortality rates for pregnant women in the initial 1976 outbreak of Ebola virus in Yambuku, Zaire, in which 9 of 82 Ebola-infected pregnant women survived—a case fatality rate of 89%. During that EVD outbreak, ten live infants were born to mothers who subsequently died of the infection. All of these children also died within 19 days [42].

The 100% maternal and infant case fatality rate that has been reported for MVD is most similar to the Ebola outbreak of 1995 in Kikwit, Zaire, in which only 1 of 15 EVD-infected women survived (case fatality rate of 95.5%). All of the pregnant women during the Kikwit EVD outbreak presented with severe hemorrhage. In addition to the maternal deaths that occurred during the Kikwit outbreak, ten women (66%) had spontaneous abortions, and one woman delivered a premature stillborn infant. Four of the pregnant women died during the third trimester of pregnancy. The single maternal survivor among this group had a curettage because of an incomplete abortion after 8 months of amenorrhea [42, 43].

The first (and only) report of the potential effect of MVD on the post-infection reproductive health of female survivors of the disease was reported from the initial outbreak of MAVN in Marburg, Frankfurt, and Belgrade in 1967 [20]. There were a total 32 persons who became infected at the three geographic locations, of whom 12 were female. Two of the 12 died, and 4 of the survivors had secondary infections that resulted in milder disease symptoms, compared with cases of primary infection. Three women who had been infected and survived became pregnant 1–2 years later. In all three cases, the pregnancy outcomes were normal. The placentas were tested for Marburg virus and were found to be negative. Umbilical cord blood was tested for antibodies to MARV and was positive for IgG but negative for IgM. When the infants were tested for MARV antibodies 1 year after birth, they were negative [20].

Because clinical disease caused by the marburgviruses and Ebola virus is clinically indistinguishable, it is reasonable to postulate that they have a similar, if not close to or even an identical, pathophysiology when affecting pregnant women and their fetuses. The first report of EVD occurring in pregnant women originated in the first reported outbreak of this disease in Zaire (now DRC) in 1976 [44]. This outbreak in the rural town of Yambuku infected a total of 316 persons, causing 280 deaths over a period of 11 weeks. There were 73 deaths among the 82 pregnant women infected with Ebola virus, a case fatality rate (CFR) of 89% [44]. Analysis of all EVD outbreaks prior to the West Africa Ebola epidemic reveals that there were 112 cases of pregnant women reported who had acquired the infection—an aggregate maternal mortality rate of 86% [11].

At the start of the West Africa epidemic and based on prior EVD outbreaks, the prognosis was considered to be so poor for pregnant women and their fetuses that it was predicted that greater than 90% of infected pregnant women and 100% of fetuses would die as a result of EVD. In an interview performed early in the outbreak with a representative from a nongovernmental organization, it was opined that the survival rate for expectant mothers was virtually zero [1]. In a report published in 2015, the probability for maternal and infant survival of EVD was summarized as follows: "Present data suggests that maternal mortality remains high (approximately 95%) and peri-natal mortality virtually 100% for infected pregnant women" [45]. Fortunately, by the close of the epidemic, the maternal mortality rate for EVD, although high, was significantly less than some had originally expected. An accurate assessment of the maternal mortality data resulting from this multinational epidemic has been made difficult by multiple factors—it was not routine practice to test infected women for pregnancy, there were infected pregnant women who did not receive care due to mobility, there were financial or social issues or the inability to reach treatment centers, case surveillance and reporting infrastructure was weakened, and many early pregnancy cases were simply missed. Within these limitations, the combined published direct mortality rates among pregnant women with EVD have been estimated to be 44% [11]. However, in addition to direct deaths caused by Ebola virus infection, many pregnant women probably died during the epidemic from indirect causes resulting from an inability to access maternal health care, diversion of already limited resources to care for persons with EVD, stigmatization and fear of attending health care facilities.

In contrast, the fetal survival rate was close to what had been expected—only one neonate is known to have survived infection. The sole surviving newborn with EVD, Baby Nubia, had received experimental treatments from Médecins Sans Frontières including ZMapp and the broad-spectrum antiviral GS-5734 outside of the clinical trial protocol; her mother had been denied access to potentially protective vaccination due to her pregnant condition and died of Ebola infection shortly after delivery [1].

The West Africa Ebola epidemic of 2013–2015, which officially infected 28,616 persons but almost certainly infected many more, resulted in a significant increase of information about filovirus infections occurring during pregnancy [46–48]. Much of these data are the subject of a multiauthored 2019 book, *Pregnant in the Time of Ebola: Women and Their Children in the 2013–2015 West African Epidemic* [48].

In addition to maternal, fetal, and infant mortalities occurring as a result of acute EVD, information regarding the subsequent effects of EVD on pregnancy and the fetus are still being analyzed, especially among female survivors and the PREVAIL Study. Fallah et al. [49] examined pregnancy outcomes in two locations (Margibi and Montserrado) for 70 female survivors of acute EVD in Liberia. Of these 70 survivors, 15 women miscarried (6 in Montserrado, 9 in Margibi); 4 neonates were stillborn (defined as fetal death ≥28 weeks' gestation, 3 in Montserrado, 1 in Margibi); and there were two EVD survivors who decided to terminate their pregnancies (both in Montserrado). Six women became pregnant within 2 months of being discharged from the Ebola treatment unit—three of these resulted in stillbirths. One additional stillbirth occurred in an EVD survivor who had conceived 6 months after recovery. All 15 miscarriages that were identified in this cohort occurred in women who became pregnant 4 months or longer after discharge. Overall the frequency of miscarriage in clinically identified pregnancies for this cohort of Ebola survivors was 22.1% (15/68), a rate slightly higher than that expected for healthy women in developed countries (between 10 and 15%) and women in West Africa (11–13%) [49].

One of the significant findings pertaining to pregnancy arising from the West Africa Ebola epidemic was the potential long-term persistence of filovirus in the tissues of women following clinical recovery from acute infection. The investigation of a family cluster of Ebola virus disease infections that occurred in Liberia provided evidence for long-term persistence of virus in some infected women [50]. Following the infection of a 15-year-old boy in Liberia with EVD in November 2015 and his subsequent death, the evaluation of other family members revealed that his 8-year-old brother had Ebola RNA in his blood, a 5-year-old brother had no evidence of infection, and a 2-month-old brother born in September 2015 had IgG antibodies to Ebola virus that were attributed to maternal transfer. The father had Ebola virus RNA in his blood and an antibody profile that was positive for Ebola-specific IgG and IgM that was consistent with previous EVD infection. The mother/wife had provided care for her adult brother in July 2014—he had died of presumptive EVD after he cared for EVD patients as a nurse's aide. Shortly after her brother died, she developed clinical illness that was compatible with EVD, but did not seek care, and had a miscarriage in August 2014. She was found to have a high titer to IgG and low titer to IgM anti-Ebola antibodies. In addition, with the results of genomic analysis, these findings indicated that the most plausible explanation for this family cluster of Ebola virus infection was that the mother/wife had survived an episode of EVD in 2014 following her acquiring it from providing care for her infected brother. She then developed persistent Ebola infection, transmitting the virus to her three family members 1 year later [16, 50].

6. Non-human primate models of Marburg virus disease

Pathological examination of the placenta and fetus and in those cases of maternal death, autopsy of the mother, have proved very helpful in understanding of the mechanisms of maternal-fetal transmission of emerging infectious diseases. This has been most recently demonstrated with the role of placental pathology in helping to understand vertical transmission of the newly emergent TORCH virus infection caused by *Zika virus* [51–54]. However, in the case of filovirus infections such as EVD and MVD, the recommendations from international organizations against pathology examination of placentas, autopsies, and fetal tissues to minimize risk of infection to healthcare workers have diminished our knowledge of the effects on pregnant women, fetuses, and neonates [11].

Experimental studies of laboratory animal infection with infectious agents can be a major source of information on the mechanisms of maternal-fetal transmission of disease, as well as the role of the placenta in vertical infections. There have been many experimental studies of infection with marburgviruses using a variety of non-human primates (NHPs)—these have included cynomolgus macaques (*Macaca fascicularis*), rhesus macaques (*Macaca mulatta*), African green monkeys (*Cercopithecus aethiops*), and squirrel monkeys (*Saimiri* sp.) [31]. Unfortunately, they have not addressed pregnancy or vertical viral transmission. There is, in addition, a paucity of information available on the effects of experimental MVD infection in non-human primates on the pathological effects on the female genital organs in nonpregnant animals, despite the performance of many autopsies.

However, some recent data are available specifically on the pathology of MVD of the female genitalia in NHPs. Four female rhesus macaques were experimentally infected via the intramuscular route with a target dose of 1000 plaque-forming units of Marburg virus/H.sapiens-tc/AGO/2005/Ang-1379v (BioSample identifier SAMN05916381), passage Vero E6p4 [55]. Microscopic examination of ovaries from three of the four MARV-infected macaques revealed degeneration and necrosis of circumferential stromal cells surrounding secondary and tertiary follicles and rare intracytoplasmic viral inclusions. In all four female macaques, immunohistochemical staining demonstrated that theca interna cells were strongly and diffusely positive for GP (Marburg glycoprotein) and VP40 (Marburg matrix protein) antigens, as well as positivity in scattered clusters of interstitial ovarian stromal cells located between the follicles. In one of the infected female macaques, there was positive staining noted in clusters of granulosa cells in secondary and tertiary follicles. Electron microscopic examination revealed viral nucleocapsids present that formed cytoplasmic tubular and granular inclusions within interstitial stromal cells and theca interna cells and the presence of mature free virus particles and in one macaque confirmed the occurrence of MARV infection in granulosa cells. The virus had also reached the fallopian tubes—all four females had positive findings of immunostaining and in situ hybridization in the epithelial cells (and stroma) of the fimbriae of the oviduct. One macaque had clusters of viral-positive smooth muscle cells in the myosalpinx. In one of the macaques, the uterus demonstrated that low to moderate numbers of vacuolated, apoptotic, and inclusion-bearing macrophages were present in the endometrial stroma; the uteri from the remaining three macaques were histologically normal. Virus was present in the uterine tissues, as evidenced by multifocal to diffuse positive immunostaining and MARV genomic in situ hybridization of the superficial endometrial stroma, and with multifocal positive staining in one of the females. Ultrastructural analysis showed small numbers of viral nucleocapsids present that formed cytoplasmic tubular and granular inclusions in several cell types, including endometrial stromal cells, fibroblasts, and endothelial cells, but not smooth muscle [55].

7. Conclusions

Marburg virus disease is a life-threatening infection to pregnant women and their infants and has fortunately been much less prevalent than its close filovirus relative, Ebola virus disease. However, mostly as a result of the West Africa Ebola epidemic, there is much more information available regarding the pathophysiology and clinical outcomes of EVD in pregnant women and their fetuses. It is likely that both the marburgviruses and Ebola virus have the same mechanism(s) of maternal-fetal transmission. Both filovirus species can persist in body tissues of survivors and be sexually transmitted. Prior to the West Africa Ebola epidemic, the case fatality rate for EVD in pregnant women varied up to greater than 90%, and all fetuses and neonates from infected women died. Fortunately, the maternal mortality rate for EVD declined during the West Africa epidemic, and as a result of the development of effective forms of therapy, the first neonatal survivor was reported. In contrast, the only reported data for maternal and neonatal survival following MVD shows a 100% mortality rate for pregnant women and their infants. Thus, based upon available, albeit limited, data, MVD has a higher case fatality rate in pregnant women than does EVD. The geographic range of MVD cases has been geographically restricted within Africa to Kenya, Uganda, DR Congo, Angola, Rhodesia, and South Africa. However, the recent announcement that the bat host for marburgviruses (*Rousettus aegyptiacus*) was found to be positive for the virus in Sierra Leone has added a potential new chapter to the risk for additional African outbreaks in a previously uninvolved part of the continent.

Author details

David A. Schwartz
Medical College of Georgia, Augusta University, Augusta, Georgia, USA

*Address all correspondence to: davidalanschwartz@gmail.com

References

[1] Schwartz DA. Clinical trials and administration of Zika virus vaccine in pregnant women: Lessons (that should have been) learned from excluding immunization with the Ebola vaccine during pregnancy and lactation. Vaccines (Basel). 2018;**6**(4):E81. DOI: 10.3390/vaccines6040081

[2] CDC. Outbreaks Chronology: Marburg Hemorrhagic Fever. 2014. Available from: https://www.cdc.gov/vhf/marburg/outbreaks/chronology.html. [Accessed: 14 May 2019]

[3] Spickler A. Ebolavirus and Marburgvirus Infections. 2016. Available from: http://www.cfsph.iastate.edu/Factsheets/pdfs/viral_hemorrhagic_fever_filovirus.pdf. [Accessed: 1 June 2019]

[4] Schindell BG, Webb AL, Kindrachuk J. Persistence and sexual transmission of filoviruses. Viruses. 2018;**10**(12):683. DOI: 10.3390/v10120683

[5] Feldmann H, Geisbert TW. Ebola haemorrhagic fever. Lancet. 2011;**377**:849-862. DOI: 10.1016/S0140-6736(10)60667-8

[6] Bebell LM, Riley LE. Ebola virus disease and Marburg disease in pregnancy: A review and management considerations for filovirus infection. Obstetrics and Gynecology. 2015;**125**(6):1293-1298. DOI: 10.1097/AOG.0000000000000853

[7] Towner JS, Amman BR, Sealy TK, Carroll SA, Comer JA, Kemp A, et al. Isolation of genetically diverse Marburg viruses from Egyptian fruit bats. PLoS Pathogens. 2009;7:e1000536. DOI: 10.1371/journal.ppat.1000536

[8] CDC. Deadly Marburg Virus Found in Sierra Leone bats. First Time this Ebola-Like Virus Identified in West Africa. 2018. Available from: https://www.cdc.gov/media/releases/2018/p1220-marburg-found-in-bats.html. [Accessed: 11 May 2019]

[9] Schnirring L. Marburg-carrying bats found in West Africa for first time. CIDRAP 2018. Available from: http://www.cidrap.umn.edu/news-perspective/2018/12/marburg-carrying-bats-found-west-africa-first-time. [Accessed: 11 May 2019]

[10] Peterson AT, Lash RR, Carroll DS, Johnson KM. Geographic potential for outbreaks of Marburg hemorrhagic fever. American Journal of Tropical Medicine and Hygiene. 2006;**75**(1):9-15. Available from: https://pdfs.semanticscholar.org/4871/a570581b7b9c441dacb68de07e3a01c5913d.pdf. [Accessed: 26 May 2019]

[11] Bebell LM. Ebola virus disease and pregnancy: Perinatal disease and transmission. In: Pregnant in the Time of Ebola: Women and their Children in the 2013-2015 West African Epidemic. Schwartz DA, Anoko JA, Abramowitz S, editors. Springer Nature, New York and Berlin. 2019. P. 53-65

[12] Spina A, Lenglet A, Beversluis D de Jong M Vernier L Spencer C, et al. A large outbreak of hepatitis E virus genotype 1 infection in an urban setting in Chad likely linked to household level transmission factors, 2016-2017. PLoS One. 2017;**12**(11):e0188240. DOI: 10.1371/journal.pone.0188240

[13] Strong A, Schwartz DA. Effects of the west African Ebola epidemic on health care of pregnant women - stigmatization with and without infection. In: Pregnant in the Time of Ebola: Women and their Children in the 2013-2015 West African Epidemic. Schwartz DA, Anoko JA, Abramowitz S, editors. Springer Nature, New York and Berlin. 2019. P. 11-30. Available from: https://link.springer.com/

chapter/10.1007/978-3-319-97637-2_2. [Accessed: 1 June 2019]

[14] Schwartz DA. All the mothers are dead – Ebola's chilling effects on the young women of one Liberian town named Joe blow In: Pregnant in the Time of Ebola: Women and their Children in the 2013-2015 West African Epidemic. Schwartz DA, Anoko JA, Abramowitz S, editors. Springer Nature, New York and Berlin. 2019. P. 251-260. Available from: https://link.springer.com/chapter/10.1007/978-3-319-97637-2_17. [Accessed: 1 June 2019]

[15] Sissoko D, Keïta M, Diallo B, Aliabadi N, Fitter DL, Dahl BA, et al. Ebola virus persistence in breast milk after no reported illness: A likely source of virus transmission from mother to child. Clinical Infectious Diseases. 2017;**64**(4):513-516. Available from: https://academic.oup.com/cid/article/64/4/513/2666520. [Accessed: 1 June 2019]

[16] Godwin CL, Schwartz DA. Uncovering more questions: Salome Karwah and the lingering impact of Ebola virus disease on the reproductive health of survivors. In: Pregnant in the Time of Ebola: Women and their Children in the 2013-2015 West African Epidemic. Schwartz DA, Anoko JA, Abramowitz S, editors. Springer Nature, New York and Berlin. 2019. P. 243-250

[17] US Army Medical Research Institute of Infectious Diseases. Mechanism of Marburg virus sexual transmission identified in nonhuman primates. ScienceDaily. 30 August 2018. Available from: www.sciencedaily.com/releases/2018/08/180830180111.htm. [Accessed: 19 May 2019]

[18] Coffin KM, Liu J, Warren TK, Blancett CD, Kuehl KA, Nichols DK, et al. Persistent Marburg virus infection in the testes of nonhuman primate survivors. Cell Host & Microbe. 2018;**24**(3):405-416. DOI: 10.1016/j.chom.2018.08.003

[19] Kissling RE, Murphy FA, Henderson BE. Marburg virus. Annals of the New York Academy of Sciences. 1970;**174**(2):932-945. DOI: 10.1111/j.1749-6632.1970.tb45614.x

[20] Slenczka W, Klenk HD. Forty years of Marburg virus. The Journal of Infectious Diseases. 2007;**196**(Suppl 2):S131-S135. DOI: 10.1086/520551

[21] Gear JS, Cassel GA, Gear AJ, Trappler B, Clausen L, Meyers AM, et al. Outbreak of Marburg virus disease in Johannesburg. British Medical Journal. 1975;**5995**:489-493. Available from: https://www.ncbi.nlm.nih.gov/pmc/articles/PMC1675587/. [Accessed: 7 May 2019]

[22] Smith DH, Johnson BK, Isaacson M, Swanapoel R, Johnson KM, Killey M, et al. Marburg-virus disease in Kenya. Lancet. 1982;**1**(8276):816-820. DOI: 10.1016/S0140-6736(82)91871-2

[23] Johnson ED, Johnson BK, Silverstein D, Tukei P, Geisbert TW, Sanchez AN, et al. Characterization of a new Marburg virus isolated from a 1987 fatal case in Kenya. Archives of Virology. 1996;**11**(Suppl.):101-114

[24] Beer B, Kurth R, Bukreyev A. Characteristics of Filoviridae: Marburg and Ebola viruses. Die Naturwissenschaften. 1999;**86**(1):8-17. DOI: 10.1007/s001140050562

[25] Nikiforov VV, Turovskiĭ I, Kalinin PP, Akinfeeva LA, Katkova LR, Barmin VS, et al. A case of a laboratory infection with Marburg fever. Zhurnal Mikrobiologii, Epidemiologii, i Immunobiologii. 1994;(3):104-106

[26] Bausch DG, Nichol ST, Muyembe-Tamfum JJ, Borchert M, Rollin PE, Sleurs H, et al. Marburg hemorrhagic fever associated with multiple genetic

lineages of virus. New England Journal of Medicine. 2006;**355**(9):909-919. DOI: 10.1056/nejmoa051465

[27] Ligon BL. Outbreak of Marburg hemorrhagic fever in Angola: A review of the history of the disease and its biological aspects. Seminars in Pediatric Infectious Diseases. 2005;**16**(3): 219-224. Available from: https://www.sciencedirect.com/science/article/pii/S1045187005000464. [Accessed: 9 May 2019]

[28] Roddy P, Thomas SL, Jeffs B, Nascimento Folo P, Pablo Palma P, Moco Henrique B, et al. Factors associated with Marburg hemorrhagic fever: Analysis of patient data from Uige, Angola. Journal of Infectious Diseases. 2010;**201**(12):1909-1918. DOI: 10.1086/652748

[29] Towner JS, Khristova ML, Sealy TK, Vincent MJ, Erickson BR, Bawiec DA, et al. Marburgvirus genomics and association with a large hemorrhagic fever outbreak in Angola. Journal of Virology. 2006;**80**(13):6497-6516. Available from: https://www.ncbi.nlm.nih.gov/pmc/articles/PMC1488971/. [Accessed: 10 May 2019]

[30] CIDRAP. Angola declares worst Marburg outbreak over. 2005. Available from: http://www.cidrap.umn.edu/news-perspective/2005/11/angola-declares-worst-marburg-outbreak-over. [Accessed: 9 May 2009

[31] Glaze ER, Roy MJ, Dalrymple LW, Lanning LL. A comparison of the pathogenesis of Marburg virus disease in humans and nonhuman primates and evaluation of the suitability of these animal models for predicting clinical efficacy under the 'animal rule'. Comparative Medicine. 2015;**65**(3): 241-259. Available from: https://www.ncbi.nlm.nih.gov/pmc/articles/PMC4485633/. [Accessed: 10 May 2019]

[32] CDC. Brief report outbreak of Marburg virus hemorrhagic fever—Angola, October 1, 2004–march 29, 2005. MMWR. Morbidity and Mortality Weekly Report. 2005;**54**(12):308-309. Available from: https://www.cdc.gov/mmwr/preview/mmwrhtml/mm54d330a1.htm. [Accessed: 10 May 2019]

[33] Jeffs B, Roddy P, Weatherill D, de la Rosa O, Dorion C, Iscla M, et al. The Medecins sans Frontieres intervention in the Marburg hemorrhagic fever epidemic, Uige, Angola, 2005. I. Lessons learned in the hospital. Journal of Infectious Diseases. 2007;**196**(Suppl 2):S154-S161. Available from: https://academic.oup.com/jid/article/196/Supplement_2/S154/858898. [Accessed: 10 May 2019]

[34] Adjemian J, Farnon EC, Tschioko F, Wamala JF, Byaruhanga E, Bwire GS, et al. Outbreak of Marburg hemorrhagic fever among miners in Kamwenge and Ibanda Districts, Uganda, 2007. The Journal of Infectious Diseases. 2011;**204**(Suppl 3):S796-S799. DOI: 10.1093/infdis/jir312

[35] Timen A, Koopmans MP, Vossen AC, Van Doornum GJ, Günther S, Van Den Berkmortel F, et al. Response to imported case of Marburg hemorrhagic fever, the Netherlands. Emerging Infectious Diseases. 2009;**15**(8):1171-1175. DOI: 10.3201/eid1508.090015

[36] CDC. Imported case of Marburg hemorrhagic fever - Colorado, 2008. Morbidity and Mortality Weekly Report. 2009;**58**(49):1377-1381

[37] Nyakarahuka L, Ojwang J, Tumusiime A, Balinandi S, Whitmer S, Kyazze S, et al. Isolated case of Marburg virus disease, Kampala, Uganda, 2014. Emerging Infectious Diseases. 2017;**23**(6):1001-1004. DOI: 10.3201/eid2306.170047

[38] WHO. Marburg Haemorrhagic Fever in Uganda – update. 2012.

Available from: https://www.who.int/csr/don/2012_10_31/en/. [Accessed: 9 May 2019]

[39] WHO. Marburg Virus Disease – Uganda. 2014. Available from: https://www.who.int/csr/don/13-november-2014-marburg/en/. [Accessed: 11 May 2019]

[40] WHO. WHO Supports Containment of Rare Virus on Uganda-Kenya border. 2017. Available from: https://www.who.int/en/news-room/detail/20-10-2017-who-supports-containment-of-rare-virus-on-uganda-kenya-border. [Accessed: 10 May 2019]

[41] WHO. Marburg Virus Disease – Uganda and Kenya. 2017. Available from: https://www.who.int/csr/don/7-november-2017-marburg/en/. [Accessed: 10 May 2019]

[42] Mupapa K, Mukundu W, Bwaka MA, Kipasa M, De Roo A, Kuvula K, et al. Ebola hemorrhagic fever and pregnancy. Journal of Infectious Diseases. 1999;**179**(Suppl. 1):S11-S12

[43] Lyman M, Mpofu JJ, Soud F, Oduyebo T, Ellington S, Schlough GW, et al. Maternal and perinatal outcomes in pregnant women with suspected Ebola virus disease in Sierra Leone, 2014. International Journal of Gynaecology and Obstetrics. 2018;**142**(1):71-77. DOI: 10.1002/ijgo.12490

[44] Report of an International Commission. Ebola haemorrhagic fever in Zaire, 1976. Bulletin of the World Health Organization. 1978;**56**(2):271-293. Available from: https://www.ncbi.nlm.nih.gov/pmc/articles/PMC2395567/. [Accessed: 10 May 2019]

[45] Black B. Principles of Management for Pregnant Women with Ebola: A Western Context. 2015. Available from: www.rcog.org.uk/globalassets/documents/news/ebola-and-pregnancy-western.pdf. [Accessed: 1 June 2019]

[46] Black BO, Caluwaerts S, Achar J. Ebola viral disease and pregnancy. Obstetric Medicine. 2015;**8**(3):108-113. DOI: 10.1177/1753495X15597354

[47] Jamieson DJ, Uyeki TM, Callaghan WM, Meaney-Delman D, Rasmussen SA. What obstetrician-gynecologists should know about Ebola: A perspective from the Centers for Disease Control and Prevention. Obstetrics and Gynecology. 2014;**124**(5):1005-1010. DOI: 10.1097/AOG.0000000000000533

[48] Schwartz DA, Anoko JN, Abramowitz S. Pregnant in the Time of Ebola: Women and their Children in the 2013-2015 West African Epidemic. New York and Berlin: Springer; 2019

[49] Fallah MP, Skrip LA, Dahn BT, Nyenswah TG, Flumo H, Glayweon M, et al. Pregnancy outcomes in Liberian women who conceived after recovery from Ebola virus disease. The Lancet Global Health. 2016;**4**(10):e678-e679. DOI: 10.1016/S2214-109X(16)30147-4

[50] Dokubo EK, Wendland A, Mate SE, Ladner JT, Hamblion EL, Raftery P, et al. Persistence of Ebola virus after the end of widespread transmission in Liberia: An outbreak report. The Lancet Infectious Diseases. 2018;**18**(9):1015-1024. DOI: 10.1016/S1473-3099(18)30417-1

[51] Schwartz DA. Viral infection, proliferation and hyperplasia of Hofbauer cells and absence of inflammation characterize the placental pathology of fetuses with congenital Zika virus infection. Archives of Gynecology and Obstetrics. 2017;**295**(6):1361-1368. DOI: 10.1007/s00404-017-4361-5

[52] Schwartz DA. Autopsy and postmortem studies are concordant. Pathology of Zika virus infection is

neurotropic in fetuses and infants with microcephaly following transplacental transmission. Archives of Pathology & Laboratory Medicine. 2017;**141**(1):68-72. DOI: 10.5858/arpa.2016-0343-OA

[53] Ritter JM, Martines RB, Zaki SR. Zika virus: Pathology from the pandemic. Archives of Pathology & Laboratory Medicine. 2017;**141**(1):49-59

[54] Rosenberg AZ, Yu W, Hill DA, Reyes CA, Schwartz DA. Placental pathology of Zika virus and microcephaly – Viral infection of the placenta induces villous stromal macrophage (Hofbauer cell) proliferation and hyperplasia. Archives of Pathology & Laboratory Medicine. 2017;**141**(1):43-48. DOI: 10.5858/arpa.2016-0401-OA

[55] Cooper TK, Sword J, Johnson JC, Bonilla A, Hart R, Liu DX, et al. New insights into Marburg virus disease pathogenesis in the rhesus macaque model. Journal of Infectious Diseases. 2018;**218**(Suppl_5):S423-S433. DOI: 10.1093/infdis/jiy367

Section 4

Immunology of Filoviruses

Chapter 4

Interaction of Ebola Virus with the Innate Immune System

Felix B. He, Krister Melén, Laura Kakkola and Ilkka Julkunen

Abstract

Ebola viruses (EBOV) are zoonotic pathogens that cause severe diseases in humans and have been responsible for several disease outbreaks over the past 40 years. Ebola virus disease (EVD) leads to death on an average of 45–50% of cases, but in some outbreaks, the figures have been higher. The largest EVD outbreak in West Africa in 2014–2015 lead to more than 28,000 cases and 11,300 fatalities. Host innate immune responses are vital in restricting the spread of viral infections including that of Ebola virus. EBOV and some other filoviruses are known to trigger uncontrolled virus replication by suppressing host innate immune responses, mainly by targeting the antiviral response through virus proteins. At least EBOV VP24 and VP35 proteins have been shown to inhibit the expression of type I and III interferon (IFN) genes as well as to inhibit IFN signaling leading to downregulated IFN-induced antiviral responses. In this review we concentrate on describing the mechanisms by which EBOV contributes to the pathogenesis of severe disease and on how the virus interacts with the host innate immune system.

Keywords: Ebola virus, filovirus, innate immunity, RIG-I pathway, MDA5 pathway, VP24

1. Introduction

Ebola virus (EBOV) belongs to the family of filoviruses which include seven viral species. Currently, eight virus types have been identified within this virus family [1]. The virus particles have a uniform diameter of 80 nm but can extend even up to 10,000 nm [2]. So far the largest outbreak of Ebola virus disease (EVD) has taken place in West Africa, in Guinea, Sierra Leone, and Liberia in 2014–2015 [3, 4]. In humans EVD is characterized by a severe disease with high fever, diarrhea and vomiting, occasionally hemorrhagic manifestations, and suppressed immune and inflammatory responses which often lead to sepsis-like symptoms and hypovolemic shock [5]. Because of its high case-fatality rate and limited treatment and vaccination options, EBOV is classified as a biothreat pathogen of category A [6] and should be handled at biosafety level 4 (BSL-4) laboratories. EBOV is also considered as one of the deadliest human pathogens and a potential bioterrorism agent [7].

EBOV infection targets many tissues and cell types leading to dysregulation of inflammatory mediators, disrupted homeostasis, and impaired host immune responses. Together with abnormalities in the coagulation and vascular system, the infection often leads to a fatal outcome in humans due to a multiorgan failure [8–10].

Invading and replicating viruses are recognized by the host via cellular pattern recognition receptors (PRRs). PRRs recognize pathogens via pathogen-associated molecular patterns (PAMPs), such as viral structural components and nucleic acids, which then activate host innate immune responses. RNA virus infection activates different PRRs like Toll-like receptors (TLRs), retinoic acid-inducible gene I (RIG-I)-like receptors (RLRs), and nucleotide-binding oligomerization domain-containing (NOD)-like receptors (NLRPs). Cell membrane-associated TLR3 and intracellular vacuole-located TLR7 and TLR8 are activated by viral dsRNA and ssRNA molecules, respectively, leading to the activation and nuclear translocation of transcription factors NF-κB, interferon regulatory factor 3 (IRF3) and IRF7 as well as MAP kinases activated transcription factors (MAPK TFs). Cytosolic RLRs, RIG-I, and melanoma differentiation-associated antigen 5 (MDA5) are activated by viral ss/dsRNA molecules leading to activation and nuclear translocation of IRF3 (and IRF7), NF-κB, and MAPK TFs [11–13]. NLRP activation, especially NLRP3, leads to the activation of the inflammasome and the production of inflammatory cytokines IL-1β and IL-18 [14].

It has been shown that the RIG-I pathway has a significant role in host innate immune responses when the pathogen is an RNA virus. RIG-I recognizes 5′-triphosphate and short ss/dsRNA structures present in genomic and replicated viral RNAs. RIG-I activates mitochondrial antiviral signaling protein (MAVS) which is located in mitochondrial membranes. MAVS triggers the activation of inhibitor kappaB kinases (IKKα/β/γ/ε) and TANK binding kinase 1 (TBK1) through tumor necrosis factor receptor-associated factor (TRAF) adaptor proteins. Activated TBK1 and IKKε then phosphorylate IRF3 [15], which forms dimers and translocates into the nucleus. At the same time, the canonical IKKα/β/γ complex activates NF-κB by phosphorylating the inhibitor of NF-κB (IκB) leading to degradation of IκB and the release and nuclear translocation of active p50-p65 NF-κB complex. NF-κB and dimerized IRF3 bind to the promoter elements of type I and type III IFN genes. This then leads to RNA polymerase II complex-initiated expression of IFN genes and secretion of type I IFN-α/β and type III IFN-λs [16]. The produced interferons are important in activating the second phase of innate immune responses in epithelial cells, fibroblasts, leukocytes, or basically any cell that has functional IFN receptors. IFN α/β and IFN-λs bind to their specific type I and type III cell surface IFN receptors (IFNAR and IFNLR, respectively) leading to activation of janus kinases (JAK) and phosphorylation and activation of signal transducers and activators of transcriptions 1 and 2 (STAT1 and STAT2). Activated STAT1-STAT2 complexes translocate into nucleus and together with IRF9 induce the expression of hundreds of host genes, which include antiviral genes like Viperin, IFITMs, PKR, OAS, and Mx genes [17].

2. Ebola virus, virus proteins, and virus replication

Single-stranded viruses with negative-sense RNA genomes can be assigned to three different subgroups whether they are multisegmented, circular, or unsegmented [18]. Unsegmented viruses belong to the order of *Mononegavirales*, and the filovirus group is one of the eight mononegaviral families [19]. Filoviruses are enveloped, non-segmented, negative-stranded RNA viruses of varying morphology. They are called filoviruses because of their filamentous particle structure [20]. Filoviruses are assigned to seven species in three genera *Cuevavirus*, *Ebolavirus* (EBOV), and *Marburgvirus* (MARV) [21]. Most of the filoviruses are human pathogens, and the diseases caused by two of these viruses, EBOV and MARV, are well-known because of their high case-fatality rate [3].

Ebola virus group includes five virus species, *Zaire ebolavirus* (ZEBOV), *Bundibugyo ebolavirus* (BEBOV), *Ivory Coast ebolavirus* (ICEBOV), *Sudan ebolavirus* (SEBOV), and *Reston ebolavirus* (REBOV). Filoviruses consist of ssRNA genomes of 19 kilobases. EBOV genome encodes eight different proteins that all have specific functions [22]. **Table 1** summarizes the major characteristics of EBOV proteins. The gene order of EBOV genome is NP, VP35, VP40, GP/sGP, VP30, VP24, and L (**Figure 1**). Nucleocapsid-associated proteins include the major nucleoprotein NP and the minor nucleoprotein VP30. Both of these proteins interact with the RNA genome and protect the viral RNA. Nucleocapsid structures also include VP35 and RNA-dependent RNA polymerase (RDRP) protein L [23]. Ribonucleoprotein complex regulates viral replication and transcription of the viral genome. The RDRP complex consists of L polymerase and VP35, the latter of which acts as a polymerase cofactor [24–26]. NP with RDRP complex catalyzes the viral genome with VP30 to initiate transcription and replication. VP40 is required for viral particle formation, and it is the major matrix protein [27]. Viral envelope glycoprotein (GP) is the only viral envelope protein, and its function is to attach the host cell surface and mediate the entry of viral nucleocapsids [28]. EBOV GP is heavily N- and O-glycosylated. On the surface of virus particles, GP is cleaved into two subunits (GP1 and GP2), and it exists as a trimeric protein complex (peplomers). In addition to full-length GP, there are several other forms of proteins encoded by the GP gene: nonstructural soluble glycoprotein (sGP) and a small soluble GP (ssGP) [29]. The functions of sGP and ssGP are presently not known, but they have been suggested to neutralize EBOV GP-specific antibodies. The viral genome encodes also VP24 which is a minor matrix protein, and its functions are dealing with virion assembly and downregulation of host innate immune responses (see below).

VP24	• Minor matrix protein, virion assembly • Inhibits type I and type III interferon (IFN) gene expression • Inhibits type I and III IFN signaling reducing the expression of IFN-induced genes (blocks STAT1/2 nuclear import)
VP30	• Minor nucleoprotein • Transcription activator
VP35	• Polymerase cofactor • Binds dsRNA and inhibits type I IFN production • Inhibits dendritic cell maturation • Blocks IKKε/TBK1 activation and IRF3 phosphorylation
VP40	• Viral matrix protein • Required in virion assembly and budding
NP	• Structural protein of nucleocapsid complex • Catalyzes viral replication and transcription of the RNA genome
GP	• Viral envelope glycoprotein • Attachment to host cell surface • Mediates virus entry • Target of anti-GP neutralizing antibodies
sGP (ssGP)	• Soluble glycoprotein (small soluble GP) • Possible decoy of anti-GP antibodies
L polymerase	• Viral RNA-dependent RNA polymerase

Table 1.
Ebola virus proteins and their functions in virus replication cycle and in host cell functions.

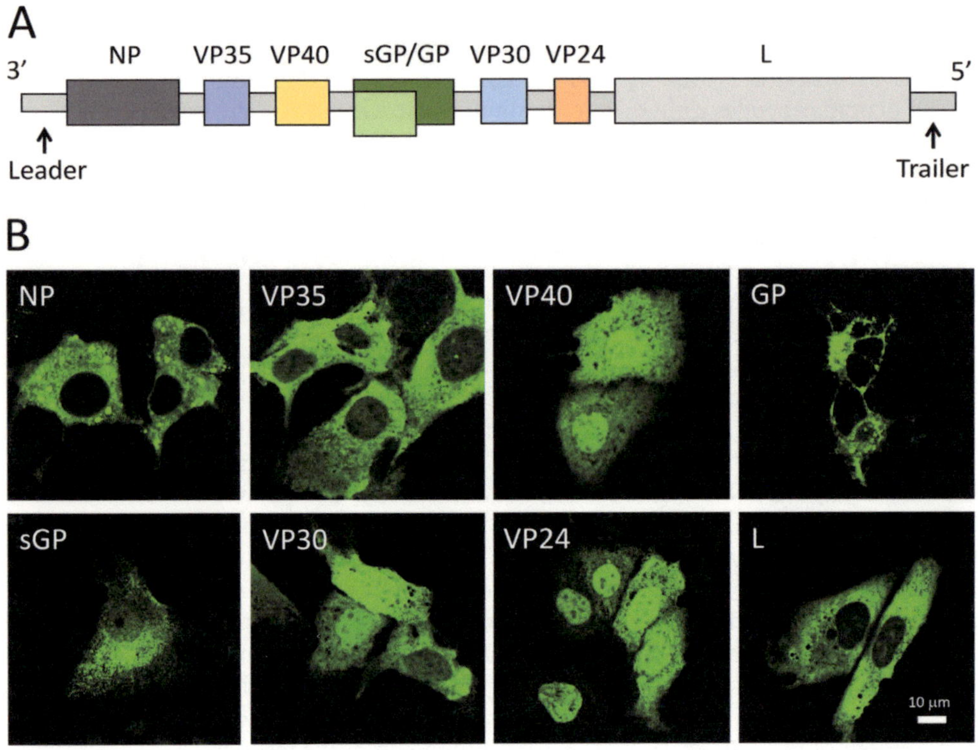

Figure 1.
Ebola virus genome structure and the expression of individual EBOV proteins in transfected cells. Panel A. EBOV genome encodes for eight different proteins, nucleoprotein (NP), viral protein 35 (VP35), VP40, secreted glycoprotein (sGP), GP, VP30, VP24, and RNA polymerase L are schematically shown. Panel B. Human hepatoma HuH7 cells were transfected with pcDNA3-His or HA-EBB expression constructs for different EBOV genes, and 24 h after transfections, the cells were stained with monoclonal anti-His (NP, VP35, VP40, GP, sGP, and VP30) or anti-HA (VP24 and L) antibodies and secondary rabbit anti-mouse immunoglobulin. Note that VP40 and especially VP24 are localized into the cell nucleus, and GP-expressing cells show significant cytotoxicity.

EBOV can infect a wide variety of cells, which may explain the ability of the virus to spread to many tissues and different types of cells. At present there is no direct evidence of one specific EBOV receptor; rather many types of molecules such as integrins, C-type lectins, and TIM-1 have been suggested to function as a cellular receptor. After attachment EBOV is endocytosed followed by a fusion of viral and endosomal membranes and release of viral nucleocapsid into the cell cytoplasm. In the cytoplasm virus-specific mRNAs are synthesized from the genomic RNA template. Viral RNA polymerase complex is responsible for the synthesis of individual mRNA molecules for each EBOV proteins. Both the transcription and translation of EBOV proteins takes place in the cell cytoplasm. Virus replication is regulated by the L polymerase, VP30, VP35, and NP followed by the assembly of viral nucleocapsid (NC) structures. GP synthesis and glycosylation occurs in the Golgi complex, and the assembly of newly produced virus particles takes place at the plasma membrane where NCs, VP40, VP24, and GP are assembled followed by virus budding from the plasma membrane [22–27].

3. Ebola virus disease (EVD)

Ebola virus disease was first recognized in 1976 simultaneously in two different geographic locations, in Sudan and in the Democratic Republic of Congo [9, 30]. The newly identified viral agent was named Ebola virus, and the symptoms resembled

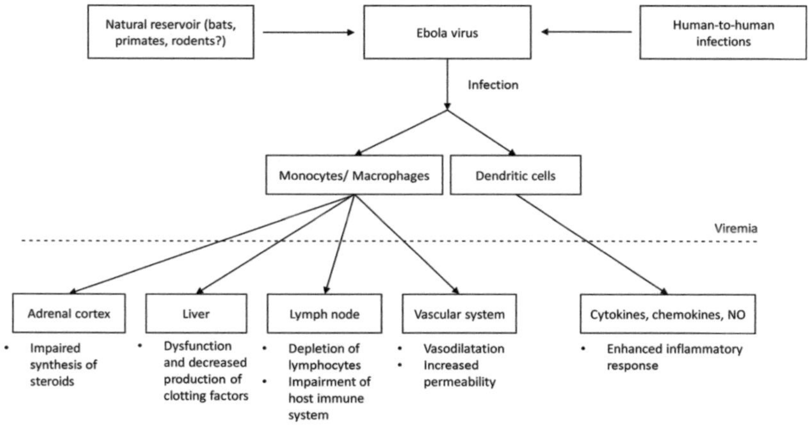

Figure 2.
Target cells and tissues infected by EBOV. Zoonotic and human-to-human transmission of EBOV through initial infection sites lead to viremia which targets the lymph nodes, liver, spleen, adrenal cortex, and vascular system. The widespread viral dissemination leads to tissue and vascular damage in these organs possibly resulting in sepsis-like state and multiorgan failure.

those of Marburg virus disease (MVD). Most human cases have been caused by the ZEBOV species, and most of the outbreaks have occurred in Central and West Africa [5]. Like in many other zoonotic diseases, EBOV is considered to have a natural reservoir in animals, but humans may also transmit the disease via blood, serum, and bodily secretions (**Figure 2**). Patients that recovered from the primary infection were found to excrete the virus for several weeks or months also via the genital tract, especially in semen [31]. Humans and possibly some other mammalian species like primates are considered as the dead-end hosts [32]. Even though there are no firm links to natural reservoirs of EBOV, many studies suggest that rodents and bats likely play a role in virus transmission [33–36]. There is strong evidence that fruit bats, in case they are in close contact with humans or when they are used as food, transmit the disease to humans. EBOV may exist silently in reservoir species and be activated through certain stimuli such as stress, coinfection, pregnancy of the carrier animals, ecological changes, and change in food habits [37, 38].

Nevertheless, the route of primary transmission from possible reservoirs to humans needs to be studied in more detail in order to prevent direct infection routes from animals to humans. During outbreaks the dominant mode of transmission is human-to-human either through mucosa or lacerations [39]. An average incubation time in EBOV epidemics with human-to-human spread has been around 9–10 days [40]. Analysis of EBOV transmission between the patient and the secondary case(s) indicates an association with an exposure to infectious bodily fluids [41]. A large meta-analysis conducted on the secondary transmissions in the same household showed that the risk of transmission was less than 1% when the person was not in direct contact with an EVD patient [42].

Once the transmission has occurred, symptoms normally arise after 4–10 days of exposure, though there is a wide variation in the incubation time ranging from 2 to 21 days [43, 44]. The typical symptoms of EVD are flu-like symptoms with fever, myalgia, and chills. Also, gastrointestinal symptoms occur as vomiting and diarrhea. After these common symptoms, the disease may rapidly evolve as hemorrhagic complications, anuria, dysthesia, and sepsis-like symptoms resulting in multiorgan failure [44, 45]. Other reported symptoms include headache, profound weakness, coughing, and rhinorrhea. Also, when systemic symptoms related to cardiovascular system occur, they often result in septic shock and edema [5, 44, 45]. Hematological changes in laboratory parameters include leukopenia, decreased neutrophil counts, and increase in liver enzymes. When the infection proceeds, patients develop thrombocytopenia, prolonged prothrombin time, and activated partial thromboplastin time. This may result in disseminated intravascular coagulation, which finally leads to a multiorgan failure and death [5]. Patients who have survived EVD were found to develop long-term symptoms and disorders such as recurrent hepatitis, myalgia, arthralgia, prolonged hair loss, psychosis, and uveitis [5, 43, 45], which in rural areas often do not receive adequate therapy.

Rapid EVD diagnosis is done by antigen detection methods (e.g., ELISA) or by the detection of viral RNA using RT-PCR techniques. High levels of viruses/viral RNA are generally seen after 48 h of clinical infection. ELISA-based EBOV-specific IgG and IgM antibody detection methods have also been developed [2]. Due to rural conditions and the fatal nature of the disease, EVD is often diagnosed based on anamnestic information and patient's symptoms [46].

Fortunately, there are promising novel therapeutic alternatives of antiviral compounds identified in *in vitro* and in animal studies [46]. Humanized monoclonal neutralizing antibody cocktails have also been used to treat EVD patients [47]. Due to the very high case-fatality rate of EVD, WHO has declared that it is ethical to use experimental drugs to treat and prevent EVD. However, to date, there are no EBOV-specific therapies that have proven their efficiency in controlled studies in humans, and thus, supportive care remains the main treatment modality for EVD patients [5, 48]. Possible future therapies would include slowing down virus replication and disease progression allowing host innate and adaptive immune responses to overcome the infection [49, 50].

Another way to approach EBOV epidemics is to use vaccines in high-risk areas. Vaccine candidates must show good efficacy in experimental EVD models [51]. Recent reviews summarize the progress made in the field of EBOV vaccines [52, 53]. Currently there are two promising vaccine candidates that have entered clinical studies: monovalent and bivalent recombinant adenovirus and VSV-based vaccines [52], the latter of which has been used in the most recent epidemic in the Democratic Republic of Congo.

4. The effect of Ebola virus infection and EBOV proteins on cytokine gene expression

Filoviruses can infect many different cell types, for example, macrophages, monocytes, dendritic cells, Kupffer cells in the liver, fibroblasts, hepatocytes, cells of adrenal gland tissue, endothelial cells, and epithelial cells (**Figure 2**) [54, 55]. In nonhuman primates it has been shown that the virus first replicates in macrophages and dendritic cells. These cells are considered to be responsible for an unbalanced immune response [55]. Studies have shown that EBOV efficiently infect these cells after they differentiate from monocytes [56–58]. Histopathological studies in human tissues have proven that macrophages are readily infected [59]. The data on cytokines and inflammatory responses show that there is a correlation between poor prognosis and intense inflammatory response characterized by excessive cytokine and chemokine production [60]. After the initial infection phase in monocyte/macrophages and dendritic cells, the virus is spreading to lymph nodes and other organs such as the liver and the spleen which takes place via the lymphatic system [54, 55]. EBOV infection in these target organs leads to strong inflammatory responses and the release of pro-inflammatory cytokines and chemokines, such as interleukin-1β (IL-1β), IL-6, IL-8, IL-10, monocyte chemoattractant protein 1 (MCP1), macrophage inflammatory protein 1α (MIP1α), MIP1β, and tumor necrosis factor (TNF) as well as to reactive oxygen species and nitric oxide [8, 61, 62].

MIP1α and MCP1 create a positive feedback loop where secreted cytokines recruit more monocyte/macrophages to the site of infection enabling EBOV to infect more target cells [55]. The infection caused by EBOV inhibits the maturation of dendritic cells and prevents antigen presentation to T cells. This event is due to EBOV infection to inhibit upregulation of CD40, CD80, CD86, and major histocompatibility complex (MHC) class II molecules [63, 64]. A commonly seen characteristic of EBOV infection is lymphopenia which occurs among $CD4^+$ and $CD8^+$ T cells and natural killer (NK) cells [65, 66]. The same effect was detected in vitro with EBOV-infected human $CD4^+$ and $CD8^+$ T cells [67]. The differences in lymphopenia profiles between the survivors and deceased patients have been linked to uncommon innate immune response and suppression of adaptive immunity [68, 69]. However, the connection between pathogenesis and the consequences of lymphopenia is presently not known. Loss of $CD4^+$ T cells may also lead to reduced production of EBOV-specific immunoglobulin M (IgM) and IgG antibodies stating that early events that occur in the immune system in EBOV infection determine the outcome of EVD [70].

The morbidity and mortality of EVD are considered to be due to a burst of immunological mediators better known as a "cytokine storm" [60, 68]. The cytokine storm is a response caused by a wide variety of infectious and noninfectious agents where they induce the production of pro- and anti-inflammatory factors usually consisting of IFNs, TNFs, interleukins, and chemokines [60, 71]. Unfortunately, the precise mechanisms triggering the cytokine storm is not known. Yet there are some studies showing that certain viruses and bacteria trigger cytokine storm through T-cell receptors and CD28 and/or by activating PAMP recognition

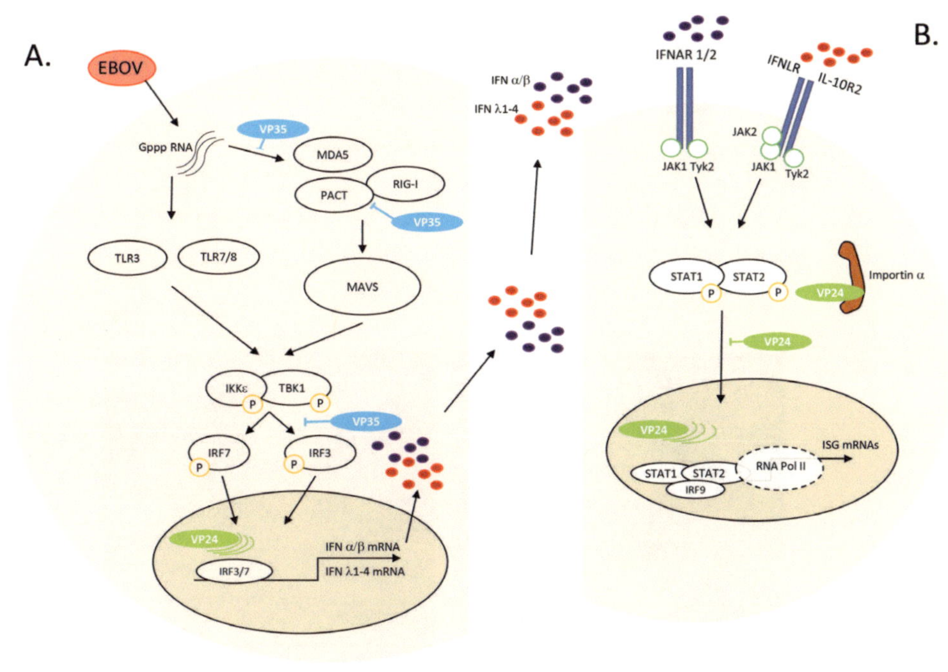

Figure 3.
Panel A. EBOV prevents type I and III IFN production and expression. Two of the eight proteins encoded by EBOV have shown inhibitory effect in previous in vitro studies: VP35 and VP24. VP35 blocks RIG-I-like signaling by binding to dsRNA or PACT and prevents IFN α/β production. It also promotes degradation of IRF3 and IRF7 by interacting with host SUMOylation process. VP35 also prevents phosphorylation of IKKε. VP24 instead inhibits IFN-λ1 gene expression downstream of IRF3. The exact mechanism is still unknown. Panel B. VP24 blocks the nuclear import of phosphorylated STAT1-STAT2 dimers by binding to importin α isoforms which limits the nuclear accumulation of activated STATs and reduces IFN-induced gene expression.

pathways [72, 73]. Since EBOV infection in macrophages and dendritic cells suppresses their cytokine and chemokine production, including that of antiviral IFNs, it is likely that the excessive production of pro- and anti-inflammatory mediators occurs in other cell types apart from macrophages and DCs [74].

The immune evasion mediated by individual EBOV proteins has also been studied. So far two of the eight or nine EBOV proteins, namely, VP24 and VP35, have been shown to interfere with the activation of innate immune responses (**Figure 3**). VP35 has been shown to inhibit the maturation of dendritic cells. It interferes with the RIG-I signaling pathway to prevent enhanced expression of MHC class I and class II and the costimulatory molecules CD40, CD80, and CD86. This leads to impaired antigen presentation to CD8+ and CD4+ T cells and to impaired T-cell activation which disrupts the linkage between innate and adaptive immune responses [75, 76]. VP35 also inhibits RIG-I signaling by preventing IFN-α/β gene expression. VP35 binds to dsRNA which inhibits the interaction of RIG-I with viral RNAs. Also, the interaction between PKR activator PACT and RIG-I is disrupted which does not allow the normal RIG-I ATPase activation to take place [77].

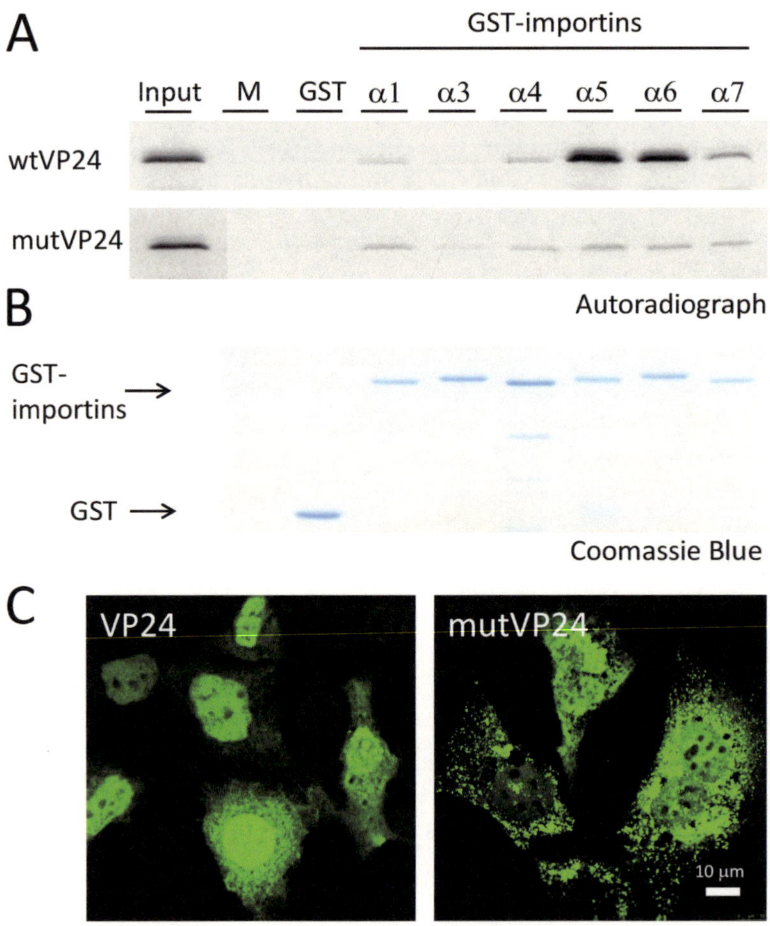

Figure 4.
Panel A. Interaction of EBOV VP24 with human importin α isoforms and intracellular location of wild-type (wt) VP24 and NLS mutant (mut) VP24. Baculovirus or E. coli-expressed GST-importin α isoforms were allowed to bind to glutathione Sepharose. In vitro-translated ^{35}S-methionine-labeled wt and mut VP24 proteins were allowed to bind to immobilized GST-importin α isoforms. NLS mutant VP24 shows clearly reduced binding to importin α molecules. Panel B shows the amount of Sepharose-bound GST-importin α molecules. Panel C shows the intracellular location of wt VP24 and reduced nuclear translocation of NLS mutant of VP24.

VP35 has also been reported to increase the SUMOylation of IRF7 by SUMO-conjugating enzyme UBC9 and SUMO E3 protein ligase PIAS1 leading to reduced transcriptional activity of IRF7 [78]. IRF7 is one of the key transcription factors regulating IFN-α/β and IFN-λ gene expression [79]. EBOV VP35 also inhibits IKKε/TBK1 kinase complex functions [80]. In addition to all the abovementioned functions, VP35 has an inhibitory effect on PKR activation that contributes to inhibition of dendritic cell maturation [61, 81].

EBOV VP24, in addition of having a role in virion assembly, is downregulating the activation of innate immune responses. In virus-infected and in VP24 gene-transfected cells, VP24 protein is expressed in the cell cytoplasm and especially in the nucleus (**Figure 1**) [82]. The expression of VP24 genes from different EBOV viruses has shown that they all inhibit RIG-I-induced IFN gene expression [83]. The analyses have been done by cotransfecting cultured cells, often human embryonal kidney cells (HEK293 cells), with the expression constructs for VP24 and activators of the RIG-I pathway (deltaRIG-I, MAVS, IKKε, or TBK1) together with IFN promoter-reporter constructs (e.g., luciferase). These analyses have revealed that VP24 is efficiently inhibiting IFN gene expression on all components of the RIG-I pathway. Interestingly, the IFN expression-inducing capacity of constitutively active form of IRF3, dimerized IRF35D construct was also inhibited by VP24. However, a mutant VP24 protein, which lacked a nuclear localization signal and was thus mostly cytoplasmic, could not interfere with RIG-I-induced IFN gene expression (**Figure 4**) [82]. This indicates that VP24 likely interferes IFN gene expression by presently unidentified mechanism in the cell nucleus.

5. Downregulation of IFN-induced antiviral activities by EBOV proteins

One of the factors dictating EBOV lethality is its ability to replicate in many cell types and evade host immune responses. There are multiple mechanisms that allow filoviruses to surpass the host innate antiviral responses, for instance, interferon-induced antiviral responses [84]. Type I and III IFNs (IFN α/β/λ) have a major role in antiviral response in viral infections [82, 85]. The activation of RLRs and TLRs and their downstream signaling cascades lead to the expression of type I and type III IFNs [11]. Type I IFNs (mainly IFN-α/β) bind to their specific cell surface receptors IFNAR1 and IFNAR2, while type III IFNs (IFN-λ1-4) have their own cell-specific receptor composed of IFNLR and IL-10R2 receptor chains (**Figure 3**). Activation of type I or type III IFN receptors leads to activation of JAK–STAT signaling pathway which ultimately leads to phosphorylation and dimerization of STAT1 and STAT2 and the expression of IFN-stimulated genes [86]. Several studies have shown that especially EBOV VP24 protein interacts with this antiviral defense system by interfering with nuclear translocation of activated STAT1-STAT2 dimers (**Figure 3B**). VP24 has a nuclear localization signal (NLS), which mediates a tight interaction with importin α molecules that mediate the nuclear translocation of nuclear-targeted proteins together with importin β. Humans have six different importin α isoforms, and VP24 is capable of binding to all importin α molecules, especially to importin α5, α6, and α7 [82]. Importin α-bound VP24 is able to prevent the interaction of STAT1-SAT2 complexes with the NLS-binding armadillo domains of importin α isoforms and thus prevent the nuclear import and subsequent STAT-induced activation of IFN-stimulated genes (ISGs). However, if the NLS of VP24 is mutated, VP24 is incapable of inhibiting importin α-STAT interaction, and IFN-induced genes are expressed normally [82].

As mentioned above, EBOV VP35 is able to inhibit dsRNA-induced PKR activation. PKR is one of the ISGs that has antiviral activity against many different viruses. EBOV GP is also able to induce cytotoxic activities in cells (**Figure 1**) even though the precise mechanisms behind this activity are present unknown.

6. Concluding remarks

Filoviruses target many cell types and tissues that regulate the activation of host immune responses and blood coagulation and hemostatic systems. Even if many of the processes in EBOV-host cell interactions have recently been revealed, there are still many open questions, e.g., by which molecular mechanisms are involved in EVD. In addition, more detailed information is needed to determine the activity of individual EBOV proteins, in addition to VP24 and VP35, on host innate and adaptive responses. Collectively, with this information it would be possible to design novel drugs or new modalities of treatment of Ebola and other filovirus infections.

7. Conclusions

Ebola virus infection is characterized by a severe infection with distorted regulation of blood coagulation and hemodynamic system and enhanced expression of inflammatory cytokines. In human infections Ebola virus targets macrophages and dendritic cells followed by systemic spread to the liver, spleen, and adrenal tissues. Individual EBOV proteins, such as VP24 and VP35, can interfere with the activation of host interferon gene expression and downregulate host antiviral responses.

Acknowledgements

The authors thank Ali Mirazimi and Helen Karlsson at Karolinska Institutet, Stockholm, Sweden, and Miao Jiang and Pamela Österlund at National Institute for Health and Welfare, Helsinki, Finland, for collaboration in the original publications. The technical assistance of Sari Maljanen is greatly acknowledged. The original research was funded by the Innovative Medicines Initiative 2 Joint Undertaking under grant agreement No. 115843. This Joint Undertaking receives support from the European Union's Horizon 2020 research and innovation program and EFPIA. The study was also supported by the Medical Research Council of the Academy of Finland (grants 252252, 256159, and 297329), the Sigrid Juselius Foundation, and the Jane and Aatos Erkko Foundation.

Conflict of interest

The authors declare no conflict of interest.

Author details

Felix B. He[1], Krister Melén[1,2], Laura Kakkola[1] and Ilkka Julkunen[1,3*]

1 Institute of Biomedicine/Virology, University of Turku, Turku, Finland

2 Expert Microbiology Unit, National Institute for Health and Welfare, Helsinki, Finland

3 Clinical Microbiology, Turku University Central Hospital, Turku, Finland

*Address all correspondence to: ilkka.julkunen@utu.fi

References

[1] Burk R, Bollinger L, Johnson JC, et al. Neglected filoviruses. FEMS Microbiology Reviews. 2016;**40**(4): 494-519. DOI: 10.1093/femsre/fuw010

[2] Rougeron V, Feldmann H, Grard G, et al. Ebola and Marburg haemorrhagic fever. Journal of Clinical Virology. 2015;**64**:111-119. DOI: 10.1016/j.jcv.2015.01.014

[3] World Health Organization. Ebola Virus Disease. 2019. Available from: https://www.who.int/ebola/en/ [Accessed: April 25, 2019]

[4] Baize S, Pannetier D, Oestereich L, et al. Emergence of Zaire Ebola virus disease in Guinea. The New England Journal of Medicine. 2014;**371**(15):1418-1425. DOI: 10.1056/NEJMoa1404505

[5] Feldmann H, Geisbert TW. Ebola haemorrhagic fever. Lancet. 2011;**377**(9768):849-862. DOI: 10.1016/S0140-6736(10)60667-8

[6] Centers for Disease Control and Prevention. Bioterrorism Agents/Diseases. 2019. Available from: https://emergency.cdc.gov/agent/agentlist-category.asp [Accessed: April 25, 2019]

[7] Borio L, Inglesby T, Peters CJ, et al. Hemorrhagic fever viruses as biological weapons: Medical and public health management. Journal of the American Medical Association. 2002;**287**(18):2391-2405

[8] Baize S, Leroy EM, Georges AJ, et al. Inflammatory responses in Ebola virus-infected patients. Clinical and Experimental Immunology. 2002;**128**(1):163-168

[9] WHO. Ebola haemorrhagic fever in Zaire, 1976. Bulletin of the World Health Organization. 1978;**56**(2):271-293

[10] Yang ZY, Duckers HJ, Sullivan NJ, et al. Identification of the Ebola virus glycoprotein as the main viral determinant of vascular cell cytotoxicity and injury. Nature Medicine. 2000;**6**(8):886-889

[11] Jensen S, Thomsen AR. Sensing of RNA viruses: A review of innate immune receptors involved in recognizing RNA virus invasion. Journal of Virology. 2012;**86**(6):2900-2910. DOI: 10.1128/JVI.05738-11

[12] Jiang M, Österlund P, Sarin LP, et al. Innate immune responses in human monocyte-derived dendritic cells are highly dependent on the size and the 5′ phosphorylation of RNA molecules. Journal of Immunology. 2011;**187**(4):1713-1721. DOI: 10.4049/jimmunol.1100361

[13] Jiang M, Österlund P, Fagerlund R, et al. MAP kinase p38alpha regulates type III interferon (IFN- λ1) gene expression in human monocyte-derived dendritic cells in response to RNA stimulation. Journal of Leukocyte Biology. 2015;**97**(2):307-320. DOI: 10.1189/jlb.2A0114-059RR

[14] Pedraza-Alva G, Pérez-Martínez L, Valdez-Hernández L, et al. Negative regulation of the inflammasome: Keeping inflammation under control. Immunological Reviews. 2015;**265**(1): 231-257. DOI: 10.1111/imr.12294

[15] Liu S, Cai X, Wu J, et al. Phosphorylation of innate immune adaptor proteins MAVS, STING, and TRIF induces IRF3 activation. Science. 2015;**347**(6227):aaa2630. DOI: 10.1126/science.aaa2630

[16] Gack MU. Mechanisms of RIG-I-like receptor activation and manipulation by viral pathogens. Journal of Virology. 2014;**88**(10):5213-5216. DOI: 10.1128/JVI.03370-13

[17] Lazear HM, Nice TJ, Diamond MS. Interferon-λ: Immune functions at barrier surfaces and beyond. Immunity. 2015;**43**(1):15-28. DOI: 10.1016/j.immuni.2015.07.001

[18] Li CX, Shi M, Tian JH, et al. Unprecedented genomic diversity of RNA viruses in arthropods reveals the ancestry of negative-sense RNA viruses. eLife. 2015;**4**:1-26. DOI: 10.7554/eLife.05378

[19] Afonso CL, Amarasinghe GK, Bányai K, et al. Taxonomy of the order *Mononegavirales*: Update 2016. Archives of Virology. 2016;**161**(8):2351-2360. DOI: 10.1007/s00705-016-2880-1

[20] Kiley MP, Bowen ET, Eddy GA, et al. Filoviridae: A taxonomic home for Marburg and Ebola viruses? Intervirology. 1982;**18**(1-2):24-32

[21] Kuhn JH, Becker S, Ebihara H, et al. Proposal for a revised taxonomy of the family Filoviridae: Classification, names of taxa and viruses, and virus abbreviations. Archives of Virology. 2010;**155**(12):2083-2103. DOI: 10.1007/s00705-010-0814-x

[22] Elliott LH, Kiley MP, McCormick JB. Descriptive analysis of Ebola virus proteins. Virology. 1985;**147**(1):169-176

[23] Volchkov VE, Volchkova VA, Chepurnov AA, et al. Characterization of the L gene and 5′ trailer region of Ebola virus. The Journal of General Virology. 1999;**80**(Pt 2):355-362

[24] Muhlberger E, Lotfering B, Klenk HD, et al. Three of the four nucleocapsid proteins of Marburg virus, NP, VP35, and L, are sufficient to mediate replication and transcription of Marburg virus-specific monocistronic minigenomes. Journal of Virology. 1998;**72**(11):8756-8764

[25] Mühlberger E. Filovirus replication and transcription. Future Virology. 2007;**2**(2):205-215. DOI: 10.2217/17460794.2.2.205

[26] Mühlberger E, Weik M, Volchkov VE, et al. Comparison of the transcription and replication strategies of Marburg virus and Ebola virus by using artificial replication systems. Journal of Virology. 1999;**73**(3):2333-2342

[27] Noda T, Sagara H, Suzuki E, et al. Ebola virus VP40 drives the formation of virus-like filamentous particles along with GP. Journal of Virology. 2002;**76**(10):4855-4865

[28] Carette JE, Raaben M, Wong AC, et al. Ebola virus entry requires the cholesterol transporter niemann-pick C1. Nature. 2011;**477**(7364):340-343. DOI: 10.1038/nature10348

[29] Mehedi M, Falzarano D, Seebach J, et al. A new Ebola virus nonstructural glycoprotein expressed through RNA editing. Journal of Virology. 2011;**85**(11):5406-5414. DOI: 10.1128/JVI.02190-10

[30] WHO. Ebola haemorrhagic fever in Sudan, 1976. Bulletin of the World Health Organization. 1978;**56**(2):247-270

[31] Deen GF, Knust B, Broutet N, et al. Ebola RNA persistence in semen of Ebola virus disease survivors—Preliminary report. The New England Journal of Medicine. 2017;**377**(15):1428-1437. DOI: 10.1056/NEJMoa1511410

[32] Groseth A, Feldmann H, Strong JE. T he ecology of Ebola virus. Trends in Microbiology. 2007;**15**(9):408-416

[33] Morvan JM, Deubel V, Gounon P, et al. Identification of Ebola virus sequences present as RNA or DNA in organs of terrestrial small mammals of the Central African Republic. Microbes and Infection. 1999;**1**(14):1193-1201

[34] Leroy EM, Kumulungui B, Pourrut X, et al. Fruit bats as reservoirs of Ebola virus. Nature. 2005;**438**(7068):575-576. DOI: 10.1038/438575a

[35] Berge T, Bowong S, Lubuma J, et al. Modeling Ebola virus disease transmissions with reservoir in a complex virus life ecology. Mathematical Biosciences and Engineering. 2018;**15**(1):21-56. DOI: 10.3934/mbe.2018002

[36] Swanepoel R, Leman PA, Burt FJ, et al. Experimental inoculation of plants and animals with Ebola virus. Emerging Infectious Diseases. 1996;**2**(4):321-325

[37] Gupta M, Mahanty S, Greer P, et al. Persistent infection with Ebola virus under conditions of partial immunity. Journal of Virology. 2004;**78**(2):958-967

[38] Strong JE, Wong G, Jones SE, et al. Stimulation of Ebola virus production from persistent infection through activation of the Ras/MAPK pathway. Proceedings of the National Academy of Sciences of the United States of America. 2008;**105**(46):17982-17987. DOI: 10.1073/pnas.0809698105

[39] Fischer R, Judson S, Miazgowicz K, et al. Ebola virus stability on surfaces and in fluids in simulated outbreak environments. Emerging Infectious Diseases. 2015;**21**(7):1243-1246. DOI: 10.3201/eid2107.150253

[40] Ajelli M, Parlamento S, Bome D, et al. The 2014 Ebola virus disease outbreak in Pujehun, Sierra Leone: Epidemiology and impact of interventions. BMC Medicine. 2015;**13**:281. DOI: 10.1186/s12916-015-0524-z

[41] Dowell SF, Mukunu R, Ksiazek TG, et al. Transmission of Ebola hemorrhagic fever: A study of risk factors in family members, Kikwit, Democratic Republic of the Congo, 1995. Commission de Lutte contre les Épidémies à Kikwit. Journal of Infectious Diseases. 1999;**179**(Suppl 1):S87-S91

[42] Dean NE, Halloran ME, Yang Y, et al. Transmissibility and pathogenicity of Ebola virus: A systematic review and meta-analysis of household secondary attack rate and asymptomatic infection. Clinical Infectious Diseases. 2016;**62**(10):1277-1286. DOI: 10.1093/cid/ciw114

[43] Kortepeter MG, Bausch DG, Bray M. Basic clinical and laboratory features of filoviral hemorrhagic fever. The Journal of Infectious Diseases. 2011;**204**(Suppl 3):S810-S816. DOI: 10.1093/infdis/jir299

[44] Jeffs B. A clinical guide to viral haemorrhagic fevers: Ebola, Marburg and Lassa. Tropical Doctor. 2006;**36**(1):1-4

[45] Hartman AL, Towner JS, Nichol ST. Ebola and Marburg hemorrhagic fever. Clinics in Laboratory Medicine. 2010;**30**(1):161-177. DOI: 10.1016/j.cll.2009.12.001

[46] Goeijenbier M, van Kampen JJ, Reusken CB, et al. Ebola virus disease: A review on epidemiology, symptoms, treatment and pathogenesis. The Netherlands Journal of Medicine. 2014;**72**(9):442-448

[47] World Health Organization. Ebola Virus Disease. 2019. Available from: https://www.who.int/medicines/ebola-treatment/ebola_drug_clinicaltrials/en/ [Accessed: April 25, 2019]

[48] Malvy D, McElroy AK, de Clerck H, et al. Ebola virus disease. Lancet. 2019;**393**(10174):936-948. DOI: 10.1016/S0140-6736(18)33132-5

[49] Feldmann H, Jones SM, Schnittler HJ, et al. Therapy and prophylaxis of Ebola virus infections. Current Opinion in Investigational Drugs. 2005;**6**(8):823-830

[50] Fischer WA 2nd, Vetter P, Bausch DG, et al. Ebola virus disease: An update on post-exposure prophylaxis. The Lancet Infectious Diseases. 2018;**18**(6):e183-e192. DOI: 10.1016/S1473-3099(17)30677-1

[51] Geisbert TW, Pushko P, Anderson K, et al. Evaluation in nonhuman primates of vaccines against Ebola virus. Emerging Infectious Diseases. 2002;**8**(5):503-507

[52] Venkatraman N, Silman D, Folegatti PM, et al. Vaccines against Ebola virus. Vaccine. 2018;**36**(36): 5454-5459. DOI: 10.1016/j.vaccine.2017.07.054

[53] Wang Y, Li J, Hu Y, et al. Ebola vaccines in clinical trial: The promising candidates. Human Vaccines and Immunotherapeutics. 2017;**13**(1):153-168. DOI: 10.1080/21645515.2016.1225637

[54] Geisbert TW, Young HA, Jahrling PB, et al. Pathogenesis of Ebola hemorrhagic fever in primate models: Evidence that hemorrhage is not a direct effect of virus-induced cytolysis of endothelial cells. American Journal of Pathology. 2003;**163**(6):2371-2382. DOI: 10.1016/S0002-9440(10)63592-4

[55] Geisbert TW, Hensley LE, Larsen T, et al. Pathogenesis of Ebola hemorrhagic fever in cynomolgus macaques: Evidence that dendritic cells are early and sustained targets of infection. American Journal of Pathology. 2003;**163**(6):2347-2370. DOI: 10.1016/S0002-9440(10)63591-2

[56] Yonezawa A, Cavrois M, Greene WC. Studies of Ebola virus glycoprotein-mediated entry and fusion by using pseudotyped human immunodeficiency virus type 1 virions: Involvement of cytoskeletal proteins and enhancement by tumor necrosis factor alpha. Journal of Virology. 2005;**79**(2):918-926. DOI: 10.1128/JVI.79.2.918-926.2005

[57] Dube D, Schornberg KL, Stantchev TS, et al. Cell adhesion promotes Ebola virus envelope glycoprotein-mediated binding and infection. Journal of Virology. 2008;**82**(14):7238-7242. DOI: 10.1128/JVI.00425-08

[58] Martinez O, Johnson JC, Honko A, et al. Ebola virus exploits a monocyte differentiation program to promote its entry. Journal of Virology. 2013;**87**(7):3801-3814. DOI: 10.1128/JVI.02695-12

[59] Zaki SR, Shieh WJ, Greer PW, et al. A novel immunohistochemical assay for the detection of Ebola virus in skin: Implications for diagnosis, spread, and surveillance of Ebola hemorrhagic fever. The Journal of Infectious Diseases. 1999;**179**(Suppl 1):S36-S47. DOI: 10.1086/514319

[60] Reynard S, Journeaux A, Gloaguen E, et al. Immune parameters and outcomes during Ebola virus disease. JCI Insight. 2019;**4**(1):1-16. pii: 125106. DOI: 10.1172/jci.insight.125106

[61] Messaoudi I, Amarasinghe GK, Basler CF. Filovirus pathogenesis and immune evasion: Insights from Ebola virus and marburg virus. Nature Reviews. Microbiology. 2015;**13**(11): 663-676. DOI: 10.1038/nrmicro3524

[62] Villinger F, Rollin PE, Brar SS, et al. Markedly elevated levels of interferon (IFN)-γ, IFN-α, interleukin (IL)-2, IL-10, and tumor necrosis factor-α associated with fatal Ebola virus infection. The Journal of Infectious Diseases. 1999;**179**(Suppl 1):S188-S191. DOI: 10.1086/514283

[63] Lubaki NM, Ilinykh P, Pietzsch C, et al. The lack of maturation of Ebola virus-infected dendritic cells results from the cooperative effect of at least two viral domains. Journal of Virology. 2013;**87**(13):7471-7485. DOI: 10.1128/JVI.03316-12

[64] Mahanty S, Hutchinson K, Agarwal S, et al. Cutting edge: impairment of dendritic cells and adaptive immunity by Ebola and Lassa viruses. Journal of Immunology. 2003;**170**(6):2797-2801

[65] Bradfute SB, Braun DR, Shamblin JD, et al. Lymphocyte death in a mouse model of Ebola virus infection. The Journal of Infectious Diseases. 2007;**196**(Suppl 2):S296-S304. DOI: 10.1086/520602

[66] Reed DS, Hensley LE, Geisbert JB, et al. Depletion of peripheral blood T lymphocytes and NK cells during the course of Ebola hemorrhagic fever in cynomolgus macaques. Viral Immunology. 2004;**17**(3):390-400. DOI: 10.1089/vim.2004.17.390

[67] Gupta M, Spiropoulou C, Rollin PE. Ebola virus infection of human PBMCs causes massive death of macrophages, CD4 and CD8 T cell sub-populations in vitro. Virology. 2007;**364**(1):45-54. DOI: 10.1016/j.virol.2007.02.017

[68] Wauquier N, Becquart P, Padilla C, et al. Human fatal zaire Ebola virus infection is associated with an aberrant innate immunity and with massive lymphocyte apoptosis. PLoS Neglected Tropical Diseases. 2010;**4**(10). pii: e837. DOI: 10.1371/journal.pntd.0000837

[69] Sanchez A, Lukwiya M, Bausch D, et al. Analysis of human peripheral blood samples from fatal and nonfatal cases of Ebola (Sudan) hemorrhagic fever: Cellular responses, virus load, and nitric oxide levels. Journal of Virology. 2004;**78**(19):10370-10377. DOI: 10.1128/JVI.78.19.10370-10377.2004

[70] Baize S, Leroy EM, Georges-Courbot MC, et al. Defective humoral responses and extensive intravascular apoptosis are associated with fatal outcome in Ebola virus-infected patients. Nature Medicine. 1999;**5**(4):423-426

[71] Tisoncik JR, Korth MJ, Simmons CP, et al. Into the eye of the cytokine storm. Microbiology and Molecular Biology Reviews. 2012;**76**(1):16-32. DOI: 10.1128/MMBR.05015-11

[72] Arad G, Levy R, Nasie I, et al. Binding of superantigen toxins into the CD28 homodimer interface is essential for induction of cytokine genes that mediate lethal shock. PLoS Biology. 2011;**9**(9):e1001149. DOI: 10.1371/journal.pbio.1001149

[73] Scherer MT, Ignatowicz L, Winslow GM, et al. Superantigens: Bacterial and viral proteins that manipulate the immune system. Annual Review of Cell Biology. 1993;**9**:101-128. DOI: 10.1146/annurev.cb.09.110193.000533

[74] Younan P, Iampietro M, Nishida A, et al. Ebola virus binding to Tim-1 on T lymphocytes induces a cytokine storm. MBio. 2017;**8**(5):1-20. pii: e00845-17. DOI: 10.1128/mBio.00845-17

[75] Yen B, Mulder LC, Martinez O, et al. Molecular basis for ebolavirus VP35 suppression of human dendritic cell maturation. Journal of Virology. 2014;**88**(21):12500-12510. DOI: 10.1128/JVI.02163-14

[76] Jin H, Yan Z, Prabhakar BS, et al. The VP35 protein of Ebola virus impairs dendritic cell maturation induced by virus and lipopolysaccharide. The Journal of General Virology. 2010;**91**(Pt 2):352-361. DOI: 10.1099/vir.0.017343-0

[77] Luthra P, Ramanan P, Mire CE, et al. Mutual antagonism between the Ebola virus VP35 protein and the RIG-I activator PACT determines infection outcome. Cell Host And Microbe. 2013;**14**(1):74-84. DOI: 10.1016/j.chom.2013.06.010

[78] Chang TH, Kubota T, Matsuoka M, et al. Ebola zaire virus blocks type I interferon production by exploiting the host SUMO modification machinery. PLoS Pathogens. 2009;**5**(6):e1000493. DOI: 10.1371/journal.ppat.1000493

[79] Österlund PI, Pietilä TE, Veckman V, et al. IFN regulatory factor

family members differentially regulate the expression of type III IFN (IFN-lambda) genes. Journal of Immunology. 2007;**179**(6):3434-3442

[80] Prins KC, Cardenas WB, Basler CF. Ebola virus protein VP35 impairs the function of interferon regulatory factor-activating kinases IKKepsilon and TBK-1. Journal of Virology. 2009;**83**(7):3069-3077. DOI: 10.1128/JVI.01875-08

[81] Feng Z, Cerveny M, Yan Z, et al. The VP35 protein of Ebola virus inhibits the antiviral effect mediated by double-stranded RNA-dependent protein kinase PKR. Journal of Virology. 2007;**81**(1):182-192. DOI: 10.1128/JVI.01006-06

[82] He F, Melén K, Maljanen S, et al. Ebolavirus protein VP24 interferes with innate immune responses by inhibiting interferon-λ1 gene expression. Virology. 2017;**509**:23-34. DOI: 10.1016/j.virol.2017.06.002

[83] Guito JC, Albarino CG, Chakrabarti AK, et al. Novel activities by ebolavirus and marburgvirus interferon antagonists revealed using a standardized in vitro reporter system. Virology. 2017;**501**:147-165. DOI: 10.1016/j.virol.2016.11.015

[84] Basler CF, Amarasinghe GK. Evasion of interferon responses by Ebola and Marburg viruses. Journal of Interferon and Cytokine Research. 2009;**29**(9):511-520. DOI: 10.1089/jir.2009.0076

[85] Schneider WM, Chevillotte MD, Rice CM. Interferon-stimulated genes: A complex web of host defenses. Annual Review of Immunology. 2014;**32**:513-545. DOI: 10.1146/annurev-immunol-032713-120231

[86] Schoggins JW. Interferon-stimulated genes: Roles in viral pathogenesis. Current Opinion in Virology. 2014;**6**:40-46. DOI: 10.1016/j.coviro.2014.03.006

Section 5

Diagnostics for Filoviruses

Chapter 5

Molecular Diagnostics of Ebola Patient Samples by Institut Pasteur de Dakar Mobile Laboratory in Guinea 2014–2016

Oumar Faye, Cheikh Tidiane Diagne, Amadou Diallo, Emily Meyer, Barre Soropogui, Gamou Fall, Cheikh Fall, N'Faly Magassouba, Lamine Koivogui, Sakoba Keita, Cheikh Loucoubar, Mamadou Diop, Manfred Weidmann, Ousmane Faye and Amadou Alpha Sall

Abstract

As part of the laboratory response to the Ebola virus outbreak in Guinea, the Institut Pasteur de Dakar mobile laboratory (IPD-ML) was set up in Donka hospital from 2014 to 2016. EBOV suspected samples collected at Ebola Treatment Centers (ETC) and from community deaths were sent daily to IPD-ML. Analysis was performed using dried oligonucleotide mixes for real-time RT-PCR designed for field diagnostic. From March 2014 to May 2015, a total of 6055 patient samples suspected for EBOV collected from seven regions of Guinea were tested by real-time RT-PCR. These patients' clinical included serum samples (n = 2537 samples) and swabs (n = 3518 samples) with positivity rates of 36.74 and 6.88% respectively. Females were significantly more affected than males with positivity rates of 22.39 and 17.22% respectively (p-value = 5.721e-7). All age groups were exposed to the virus with significant difference (p-value <= 2.2e-16). The IPD-ML contributed significantly to the surveillance and patient management during the EBOV outbreak in Guinea. Furthermore, dried reagents adapted for field diagnostic of EVD suspect cases could be useful for future outbreak preparedness and response.

Keywords: Ebola disease virus, West-Africa epidemic, mobile laboratory deployment, social benefits

1. Introduction

Ebola virus (EBOV) belongs to the family *Filoviridae*, genus Filovirus. *Filoviridae* are non-segmented negative RNA viruses belonging to the order of *Mononegavirales* together with the families *Paramyxoviridae* and *Rhabdoviridae*. Ebola virus disease (EVD) is caused by five species of the genus Ebolavirus represented by Ebola virus (EBOV), Reston virus (RESTV), Sudan virus (SUDV), Bundibugyo virus (BDBV),

 IntechOpen

Tai Forest virus (TAFV). TAFV has been associated with only one human case [1]. RESTV has only been found in non-human primates (NHP) and was found in swine suffering from porcine reproductive and respiratory disease syndrome [2].

The natural hosts of the EBOV remain unknown. However frugivorous bats of the family *Pteropodidae* are the most likely reservoir. Humans are infected with EBOV through direct contact with blood, secretions, organs or body fluids of diseased or dead animals found in the rainforest or most likely during slaughter of infected animals such as chimpanzees, gorillas, frugivorous bats, monkeys, duikers or porcupines. Human-to-human transmission is then achieved through direct contact with the secretions or biological fluids of infected persons. In hospitals and communities' cases of infections through contact with the patients and during funerals were described [3, 4]. Sexual transmission has also been documented and the virus can be isolated in the seminal fluid after several weeks of convalescence [5].

Since the discovery of EVD in 1976 in Nzara (now South Sudan) and Yambuku (Democratic Republic of the Congo (DRC)) close to the Ebola River [6], EBOV outbreaks were sporadically reported in Eastern and Central Africa from 1976 to 2014 in five countries: DRC, Sudan, Gabon, Uganda and Congo. More than 2000 cases have been reported with over 1500 deaths. EVD therefore appeared mostly geographically limited to remote villages in Central Africa until the 2014–2016 outbreak in West Africa [7–9].

In February 2014, Guinea recorded numerous cases of fatal fever in the south of the country. In March 2014, a local team conducted a first investigation in the Guinea Forest region, particularly in the prefectures of Macenta, Gueckedou, Kissidougou and Nzerékoré to collect blood samples from suspect cases of hemorrhagic fever patients. Thirty-three blood samples were sent to the Institute Pasteur of Lyon, France for laboratory investigation.

Since biosecurity concerns by airlines, obstructed air transport of more samples from Guinea to Senegal a request was issued by the Guinean Minister of Health to the WHO for the deployment of a team of the Institut Pasteur of Dakar (IPD) to Guinea to support diagnostics of the suspected hemorrhagic fever cases on March 20, 2014. On 22 March 2014 first laboratory results by the Institut Pasteur de Lyon, in France confirmed EVD cases in Guinea. The Institut Pasteur Dakar Mobile Laboratory (IPD-ML) was deployed on 23 March 2014, to the Donka hospital in Conakry and tested a first positive sample on the same day. Here, we present a summary of the laboratory's activities between March 23, 2014 and May 31, 2015 using field-based sensitive and/or rapid molecular diagnostics tools.

2. Material and methods

2.1 Organization of the laboratory

The IPD-ML was set up at Donka hospital in the Infectious Disease Department. It was organized in pre-analytical, analytical and post-analytical phases as described previously [10].

2.2 Sample collection

Clinical samples were collected at the MSF isolation ward by personnel wearing personal protective equipment (PPE) including a surgical mask, cap, shield or goggles, gown, apron, gloves (two pairs) and boots. Swab samples (nasal and oral) were collected using cotton tipped applicators (Deltalab, Spain). Whole blood samples were collected using EDTA and serum vacutainer tubes. For transport, tubes were disinfected with a 0.5% hypochlorite solution and put in triples packages bags. An Ebola investigation request form was also filled out and sent with sample to the laboratory.

2.3 Sample handling and RNA extraction

Collected samples were manipulated at IPD-ML by personnel wearing Tyvek suits, googles and gloves. Samples were inactivated in a class II biosafety cabinet (BDK Luft, Genkingen, Germany) using QIAamp viral mini kit as recommended by the supplier. Then, RNA extraction was performed in a class II biosafety cabinet (Nuaire, Minnesota, USA) and eluted in 50 μl of buffer. All waste material was treated with 1% Incidin (Ecolab, Germany) solution and incinerated on the same day.

2.4 RT-PCR diagnostic assays

RNA was detected using the quantitect RT-PCR Master Mix Probe kit (Qiagen). Briefly, 5 μl of RNA was added to 20 μl of master mix containing 2x QuantiTect Probe RT-Master Mix buffer and dried oligonucleotide mixes (Roboscreen, Jena, Germany) prepared in 4x and 10x reactions as described [11]. The real time PCR assay was performed using a Smartcycler thermocycler (Cepheid, Sunnyvale, CA). The thermal profile used was a reverse transcription for 10 min at 50°C, 15 min at 95°C for reverse transcriptase inactivation and DNA polymerase activation followed by 45 amplification cycles of 5 sec at 95°C and 50 sec 60°C (annealing-extension step).

The samples were considered positive if there was an apparent logarithmic phase in the amplification curve with a Ct value of <38. For Ct values between 38 and 42, the samples were considered suspect and undetermined and negative if there was no apparent logarithmic amplification.

2.5 Data management and statistical analysis

Patient results were recorded in a database including patient ID, date of sample collection and laboratory results. Daily, the database was sent to the ETC, the WHO and the Guinean MoH for rapid care of the patients and an update of the EVD response.

The statistical analyses were performed using the R statistical software (version 3.3.2) [12]. All calculated p-values were results of Fisher's Exact Test with a two-sided alternative hypothesis (testing for inequality).

3. Results

The algorithm for laboratory testing is presented in **Figure 1**. The IPD-ML was operational within 1 hour after the arrival in Guinea and gave results of suspected EVD cases in less than 3 hours from the time of sample receipt. From March 2014 to May 2015, a total of 6055 patient samples suspected for EBOV (53% of the total of samples tested in Guinea) were tested by the IPD-ML setup in Donka hospital, Guinea, of which 1157 tested positive by real time RT-PCR. Among the 6055 samples, 7 were EVD suspect cases from Liberia received at the IPD-ML on March 29, 2014, of which two tested positive for EBOV, confirming the first circulation of the virus in this country. The clinical specimens included mainly serum samples (n = 2537 samples) and swabs (n = 3518 samples) with positivity rates of 36.74 and 6.88% respectively (**Table 1**).

Figure 2 shows the geographical distribution of patient samples tested at IPD-ML. Overall, most of the samples tested were from Lower Guinea regions: Conakry (70%), Coyah (6.42%), Dubreka (5.38%), Forecariah (5.07%), Kindia (3.12%), and Boffa (2.59%). Furthermore, we also tested patient samples collected from the remaining regions of the country: Middle Guinea, Upper Guinea and Forest Guinea.

Analysis of all samples tested by sex, suggests a statistically significant difference between the females (n = 2608 samples) and males (n = 3397 samples) with positivity rates of 22.39 and 17.22% respectively (p-value = 5.721e-7). Analysis by sex of samples collected in Conakry, showed statistically significant difference between the females (n = 1550 cases) and males (n = 2169 cases) with positivity rates of 16.1 and 12.7% respectively (p-value = 0.01231). Furthermore, the distribution of EVD cases by age of samples collected in the Conakry region showed that all age groups were exposed to the virus with significant difference (p-value <= 2.2e-16). Patients aged 50 years and over seemed to be less affected by the outbreak.

Analysis of alive suspect EVD patients by sex show a total of 1111 females versus 1415 males tested (serum patients); for these patients 41.3% (459/1111) of females and 33.4% (472/1415) of males were tested positive with significant difference of

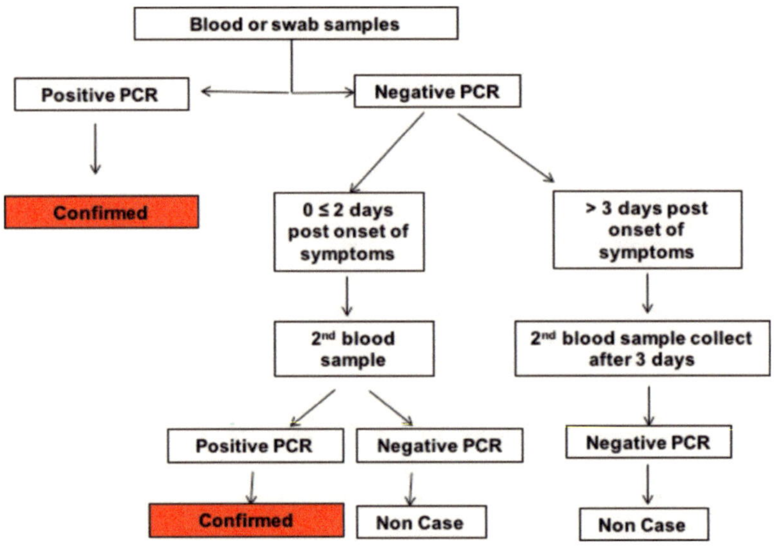

Figure 1.
Diagnostic algorithm for IPD - ML testing.

Samples source	Tested	Positives/negatives
Blood samples	2537	932/1605
Swab samples	3518	242/3276
Total	6055	1174/4881

Table 1.
Samples tested and lab results from March, 23, 2014, to May 31, 2015.

infection between the two genders (p = 4.615e-5). Females exhibited a higher ratio of infection than males during the period of study.

Analysis of alive patients by age show significant difference of infection in terms of age group with a higher rate of infection for people aged between 35 and 49 years (p-value = 0.01704) (**Table 2**).

Figure 3 shows EVD cases admitted to the ETC analyzed by IPD-ML between March 2014 and May 2015. The number of confirmed EBOV cases was almost the same per month between March and July 2014 with a total of 34.22% (128/374) confirmed cases with an average of 26 positives cases by month, and peaked in December 2014 with 253 confirmed cases.

Figure 4 and **Table 3** represent swab samples collected from deceased analyzed by month and age. Out of the 3518 swab tests performed, 242 were tested EBOV

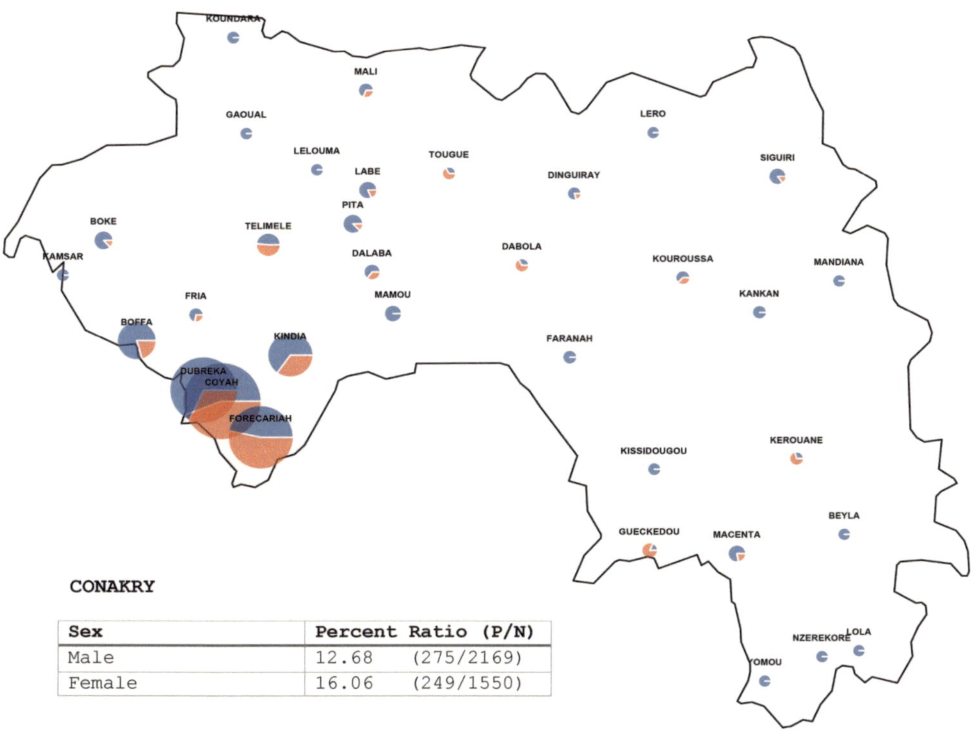

Figure 2.
Outbreak distribution map. Geographic mapping of the distribution of the epidemic throughout the country of Guinea with the exception of its capital, Conakry. Red and blue colors represent positives and negatives cases respectively. Because about two thirds (4285/6055) of all tested patients resided in Conakry, an extra table represents numbers tested and confirmed cases in the Conakry region. Inclusion of these data throws the proportion of the remaining pie charts off balance.

Age group	Positive	Negative	Ratio (P/N)	P-value
[−19]	186	323	0.57585	0.01704
[20–34]	330	612	0.53922	
[35–49]	240	325	0.73846	
[50+]	139	268	0.51866	

Table 2.
Distribution of patients (alive) by age group.

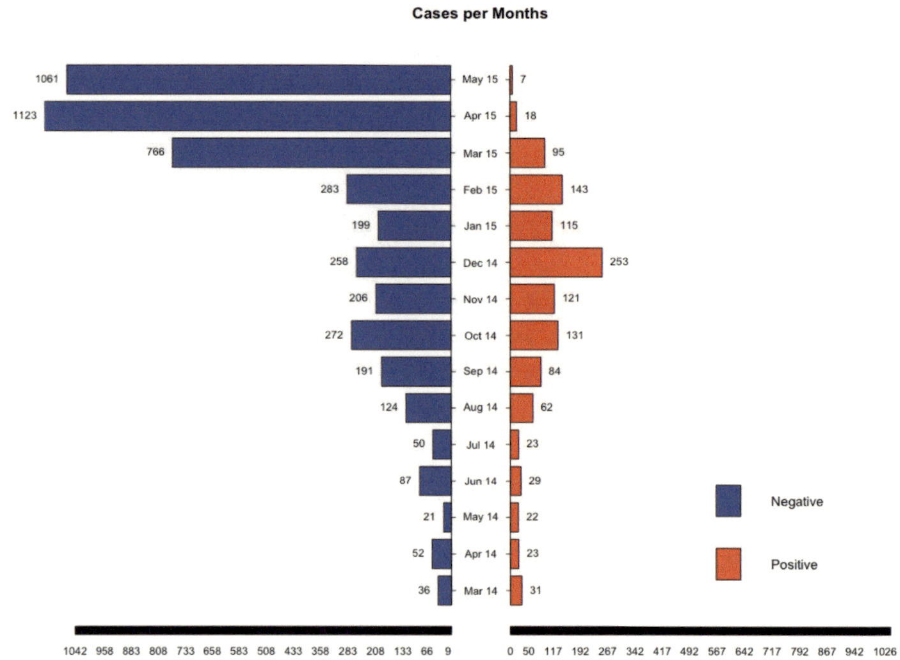

Figure 3.
Number of cases per months. The horizontal bar plot shows the number of people that were tested every month from January 2014 to May 2015. Red and blue bars represent positive and negative cases respectively.

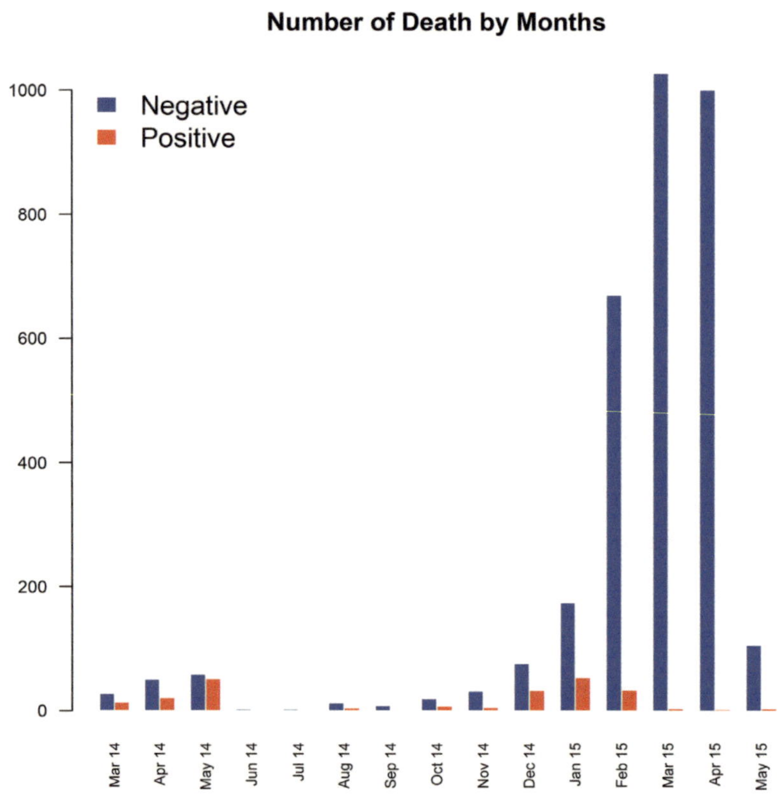

Figure 4.
Number of deaths per months. The bar plot classifies all the defunct tested patients through the months and segregates the patients by the result of their tests.

Age group	Female	Male	Ratio (M/F)	P-value
[−19]	21	19	0.90476	0.9952
[20–34]	33	28	0.84848	
[35–49]	35	32	0.91429	
[50+]	32	27	0.84375	

Table 3.
Distribution of death by Ebola per age group.

positive i.e. the cause of death had been EVD against 3276 patients that died of other causes. However, analysis of the 242 aforementioned patients grouped by age shows that there is not enough evidence to correlate deaths caused by EBOV to gender (p-value = 0.9952).

3.1 Need for rapid and portable assay for Ebola diagnostics

As in previous epidemics contacts of Ebola patients or deaths in West-Africa were found to feel helpless while fearing to die a premature death, to mourn the loss of relatives and friends and to lose the trust in others. Especially during the waiting time for the test result, they feel helpless and hopeless [13].

Long periods of waiting for the test result, enhanced a high social burden for the affected communities because of stigmatization: "When the burial team lead told [the relatives] that it could take between 2-21 days before they would know the test results, some relatives complained about the delay, noting: "the whole time, the stigma on you" [5].

In Liberia, there was a big fear among the communities to be erroneously quarantined for a non-Ebola illness so people became reluctant to search health-service when they experienced symptoms. Additionally, there was a fear of an entire households being stigmatized with Ebola and quarantined whenever deaths occurred which were most likely to be due to other diseases. Similar responses were reported from the EVD outbreak in Kikwit in 1995 and in Gulu 2001 [14, 15].

Lacking definite EVD confirmation or exclusion, the community started to hide deaths and performed secret burials in order to avoid inappropriate stigmatization and quarantine. Receiving a negative test result freed families from stigmatization due to an Ebola case.

Communities began demanding a timelier return of test results and specifically demanded a rapid diagnostic test: "I suggest that the government improve the system. People will die at home. That will always happen. But let us say, if in 2- or 3-hours' time, if government able to tell you that this is Ebola body or not Ebola body that will be very fine." (Community member FGD, Site B) [5].

Rapid point of care assays like the highly sensitive and specific RPA used in Guinea shorten the burden of emotional distress by significantly decreasing the amount of waiting time until the Ebola status is assessed.

A quicker return of results also shortens the time of inappropriate quarantine and facilitates contact tracing efforts. It counters low acceptance of testing for EVD which risks underdiagnosing EVD patients thereby facilitating spread of disease by continuous contact with other community members [5]. Rapid diagnostic tests are a key tool for providing the appropriate care for patients, according to the Ebola Response Anthropology Platform [16].

3.2 Use of recombinase polymerase amplification

The EBOV RT-RPA was successfully used in a campaign to roll back EVD cases in western parts of Conakry following an upsurge of EVD cases connected to non-reporting, reticence, and transmission chains connected to funeral rites toward the end of [17]. Mobile suitcase labs using RT-RPA tested oral swabs from all deceased at the morgue in Matoto in March and April 2015. Results were provided 30–40 min after receipt of samples to the safe and dignified burial (SDB) teams.

Altogether the suitcase based RT-RPA assay for the detection of EBOV in saliva samples proved to be very efficient and as sensitive and specific as real time PCR. The combination of SPEED Extract extraction in a hard plastic glovebox and RT-RPA in a suitcase using RPA pellets which already contained primers and probe allowed biosafe handling of samples, reduced time to result and allowed a large turnover in very simple settings [18].

There was no concomitant study to measure the impact of the RPA deployment. However the joint IPD-guinea team noticed this strategy of lowering the time to results successfully contributed to the reduction of the population reluctances to be tested. When knowledge spread in Matoto about the fast time to result for the obligatory screening of deceased, SDB teams were suddenly actively addressed and directed to deceased to take samples in order to clear bodies for traditional burials, essentially changing the behavior of the local population.

The RPA assay was deployed not only in Conakry but also during campaigns organized by the coordination committee for active search of Ebola suspected cases in the Forécariah, Coyah, Dubréka and Boké prefectures. During these campaigns, 2509 samples were tested.

The end of the Ebola epidemic was declared by the WHO on December 29, 2015. However due to the persistence of the virus in survivors, WHO recommended to strengthen the surveillance in the whole country for three additional months. Hence, a lab deployment strategy was set up in the Guinea to screen all Ebola suspected cases samples collected in the health care and community death. Then mobile laboratory based on the RPA assay was recommended by the "Coordination Nationale de Riposte au virus Ebola" to continue the real time monitoring of Ebola virus due to the rapidity and user-friendly of the assay. On 17 March 2016, the RPA system allowed the detection of the two last Ebola cases reported in Guinea, in the Nzérékoré forest area of the country [19].

4. Discussion

The use of mobile laboratories is crucial for rapid management and control of epidemics in infrastructure poor settings. During the EVD outbreak in West Africa, several mobile laboratories were deployed in the countries most affected by the deadly virus, i.e. Sierra Leone, Liberia and Guinea. In this context, the IPD deployed a mobile laboratory in Conakry, Guinea, at the Donka Hospital. Overall, a total of 4881 samples of EVD-suspect patients including live and community deaths were analyzed between March 2014 and May 2015 with 1174 confirmed positives for EBOV.

Epidemics prior to 2014 had been reported in rural areas only [9, 20]. The IPD-ML tested samples collected from all the four natural regions of Guinea. The majority of the confirmed cases tested were collected toward the end of 2014 in the Conakry region. This was due to movements of EVD cases inside a densely populated area combined with ignorance toward the disease by the population in general and in particular by medical staff although EVD had been ongoing in the country for months.

The results of the IPD-ML were systematically sent out 3 hours after samples receipt at the hospital Donka Ebola treatment center managed by Médecins Sans Frontières. Patients which tested positive were placed in the isolation zone for better care and to avoid contamination of others.

Depending on the development of the disease, the viral genome can be detected at day 2 or 3 after the onset of the disease until about day 10, and IgM and IgG can be detected at about the same time after the onset of the disease (8–10 days) [21]. Therefore, in the first 3 days of illness, and beyond 10 days after the beginning of the disease, molecular testing cannot detect the virus genome, which can lead to false negatives. Therefore, RT-PCR should be repeated for early samples taken up to 72 hours after onset of disease [22, 23]. Patients negative in the initial test therefore were observed for 48 hours in a separate zone and a second control test had to score negative before they were released.

Furthermore, for Ct values ranging between 38 and 42, the patient was also considered as a suspected case and a control test was recommended to the ETC. The real time RT-PCR method used by IPD-ML was very sensitive with a detection limit of 10 copies of RNA [18, 24, 25].

In addition, we carried out studies to improve our diagnostic platform deployed by the IPD-ML. In the face of an upsurge of EBOV cases in Conakry and transmission of the virus via funeral rites in 2014, we developed a rapid isothermal test for rapid detection of the virus in 10–15 min [18]. This method allowed rapid rendering of results and secure burial of deaths, thus contributing to a significant reduction of the transmissions of the virus during funeral rites and a reduction of social reluctance to submit samples often reported due to the expectation of the results and the consequent impact on burial rites.

It is important to note that in Conakry, where most tested patients resided, women had a significant higher infection rate which can be attributed to gender-related risk factors. The Guinean societal and organizational culture holds women responsible for nursing and caring for the patients. In an attempt to fulfill their gender roles, women were left more exposed to the virus [26].

The major challenge encountered during this deployment was the electricity supply, which can have an impact on the storage of reagents and the time to results. During the IPD-ML deployment in Guinea, these obstacles were overcome. A generator of 10 KVA was installed which supported the PFHG laboratory building. In the event of a breakdown of our generator, our diagnostic platform composed of a class III cabinet glovebox, a centrifuge, a Smart Cycler and other small bench-top equipment was powered by a system of batteries coupled with solar panels. Moreover, the use of freeze-dried primers and probes with good performances at temperatures of 40°C relieved us of energy problems.

In addition, it is important to have a differential diagnosis approach in the event of an outbreak for rapid management of non-EBOV patients. Indeed, the signs of EBOV are often similar to certain diseases such as malaria, typhoid fever, dengue that co-circulate in the same geographical areas [27].

During the 2014–2015 EVD outbreak in Guinea, the mobile laboratory running the Ebola RPA assay was run by local laboratory technicians, a sustainable option which provides local capacity for potential future outbreaks. The redeployment and strategic placement of this RPA instrument to complement EVD isolation facilities throughout the country has strengthened preparedness and response capabilities for future EVD outbreaks in Africa, particularly in West Africa [26].

The development of portable mobile platform is crucial for rapid epidemic management in resource-poor regions. The lessons learned during the Ebola epidemic, in particular the development of new equipment and reagents, will allow better management of future epidemics.

Acknowledgements

We would like to thank the Coordination Nationale de Lutte contre la Maladie à Virus Ebola (CNLEB), WHO, Médecins Sans Frontières and other partners involved in EVD outbreak responses and control. We would also like to acknowledge Hadja Aissatou Bah, Amadou Doré, Fodé Kourouma, Moussa Condé, Eugène Kolié, Mamadou Lamine Keita, Alpha Mamadou Baldé, Ibrahima Khalil Balé, Jacob Camara and Fanta Berrete for excellent technical expertise.

Conflict of interest

No conflict of interest for any of the authors declared.

Funding statement

This work was supported by the Fondation Institut Pasteur de Dakar, and the Welcome Trust programme: Research for Health in Humanitarian Crises (R2HC) grant 13,376, "Point-of-care diagnostic testing for Ebola virus disease in Ebola treatment centres".

Author details

Oumar Faye[1], Cheikh Tidiane Diagne[1], Amadou Diallo[2], Emily Meyer[1], Barre Soropogui[3], Gamou Fall[1], Cheikh Fall[1], N'Faly Magassouba[3], Lamine Koivogui[4], Sakoba Keita[5], Cheikh Loucoubar[2], Mamadou Diop[2], Manfred Weidmann[6*], Ousmane Faye[1] and Amadou Alpha Sall[1]

1 Arbovirus and Viral Hemorrhagic Fever Unit, Institut Pasteur de Dakar, Dakar, Senegal

2 Biostatistics, Bioinformatics and Modeling Unit, Institut Pasteur de Dakar, Dakar, Senegal

3 Laboratory for Hemorrhagic Fevers of Guinea, Conakry, Guinea

4 National Public Health Institute, Conakry, Guinea

5 Ministry of Health, Conakry, Guinea

6 Institute of Aquaculture, University of Stirling, Stirling, United Kingdom

*Address all correspondence to: m.weidmann@stir.ac.uk

References

[1] Le Guenno B, Formenty P, Wyers M, Gounon P, Walker F, Boesch C. Isolation and partial characterisation of a new strain of Ebola virus. Lancet. 1995;**345**(8960):1271-1274

[2] Barrette RW, Metwally SA, Rowland JM, Xu L, Zaki SR, Nichol ST, et al. Discovery of swine as a host for the Reston ebolavirus. Science. 2009;**325**(5937):204-206

[3] Victory KR, Coronado F, Ifono SO, Soropogui T, Dahl BA, Centers for Disease Control and Prevention (CDC), et al. Ebola transmission linked to a single traditional funeral ceremony—Kissidougou, Guinea, December, 2014-January 2015. Morbidity and Mortality Weekly Report. 2015;**64**(14):386-388

[4] Victory KRCF, Ifono SO, Martel LD, Keita S, Dahl BA. Unsafe burials: Challenge to controlling local Ebola outbreaks in Guinea 2015-2016. Journal of Epidemiology and Preventive Medicine. 2016;**2**(2):117

[5] Abbate JL, Murall CL, Richner H, Althaus CL. Potential impact of sexual transmission on Ebola virus epidemiology: Sierra Leone as a case study. PLoS Neglected Tropical Diseases. 2016;**10**(5):e0004676

[6] Breman JG, Heymann DL, Lloyd G, McCormick JB, Miatudila M, Murphy FA, et al. Discovery and description of Ebola Zaire virus in 1976 and relevance to the West African epidemic during 2013-2016. The Journal of Infectious Diseases. 2016;**214**(suppl 3):S93-S101

[7] Chippaux JP. Outbreaks of Ebola virus disease in Africa: The beginnings of a tragic saga. The Journal of Venomous Animals and Toxins Including Tropical Diseases. 2014;**20**(1):44

[8] Weyer J, Grobbelaar A, Blumberg L. Ebola virus disease: History, epidemiology and outbreaks. Current Infectious Disease Reports. 2015;**17**(5):480

[9] Cenciarelli O, Pietropaoli S, Malizia A, Carestia M, D'Amico F, Sassolini A, et al. Ebola virus disease 2013-2014 outbreak in west Africa: An analysis of the epidemic spread and response. International Journal of Microbiology. 2015;**2015**:769121

[10] Faye O, Fall G, Soropogui B, Koivogui L, Magassouba N, Weidmann M, et al. Deployment of the Institut Pasteur de Dakar team to Guinea in the Ebola virus Disease outbreak in West-Africa 2014-2016. Clinical Microbiology and Infectious Diseases. 2016;**1**(4)

[11] Weidmann M, Faye O, Faye O, Abd El Wahed A, Patel P, Batejat C, et al. Development of mobile laboratory for viral hemorrhagic fever detection in Africa. The Journal of Infectious Diseases. 2018;**218**(10):1622-1630

[12] Team RC. R: A Language and Environment for Statistical Computing. Vienna, Austria: R Foundation for Statistical Computing; 2014

[13] Locsin RC, Matua AG. The lived experience of waiting-to-know: Ebola at Mbarara, Uganda—Hoping for life, anticipating death. Journal of Advanced Nursing. 2002;**37**(2):173-181

[14] De Roo A, Ado B, Rose B, Guimard Y, Fonck K, Colebunders R. Survey among survivors of the 1995 Ebola epidemic in Kikwit, Democratic Republic of Congo: Their feelings and experiences. Tropical Medicine and International Health : TM & IH. 1998;**3**(11):883-885

[15] Okware SI, Omaswa FG, Zaramba S, Opio A, Lutwama JJ, Kamugisha J,

et al. An outbreak of Ebola in Uganda. Tropical Medicine and International Health : TM & IH. 2002;**7**(12):1068-1075

[16] Available from: http://www.ebola-anthropology.net/wp-content/uploads/2015/07/FINAL-Report-to-Liberia-MoH-Understanding-Why-Ebola-Deaths-Occur-at-Home-Liberia.pdf

[17] Migliani R. 3 ans après: Le point sur la dynamique de L' epidemie Ebola 3ans après: les grandes questions I; 08.11.2016; Institut Pasteur -Amphithéâtre Jacob25 -28 rue du Dr Roux, 75015 Paris; 2016

[18] Faye O, Faye O, Soropogui B, Patel P, El Wahed AA, Loucoubar C, et al. Development and deployment of a rapid recombinase polymerase amplification Ebola virus detection assay in Guinea in 2015. Euro Surveillance. 2015;**20**(44)

[19] WHO. Ebola Situation Report. 2016. Available from: http://apps.who.int/ebola/current-situation/ebola-situation-report-30-march-2016

[20] Lamunu M, Olu OO, Bangura J, Yoti Z, Samba TT, Kargbo DK, et al. Epidemiology of Ebola virus disease in the Western area region of Sierra Leone, 2014-2015. Frontiers in Public Health. 2017;**5**:33

[21] Ksiazek TG, Rollin PE, Williams AJ, Bressler DS, Martin ML, Swanepoel R, et al. Clinical virology of Ebola hemorrhagic fever (EHF): Virus, virus antigen, and IgG and IgM antibody findings among EHF patients in Kikwit, Democratic Republic of the Congo, 1995. The Journal of Infectious Diseases. 1999;**179**(Suppl 1):S177-S187

[22] Organization WH. Laboratory Diagnosis of Ebola Virus Disease. Geneva, Switzerland: World Health Organization; 2014

[23] Centers for Disease Control and Prevention (CDC). Guidance for Collection, Transport and Submission of Specimens for Ebola Virus Testing. 2015

[24] Weidmann M, Muhlberger E, Hufert FT. Rapid detection protocol for filoviruses. Journal of Clinical Virology. 2004;**30**(1):94-99

[25] Jaaskelainen AJ, Sironen T, Diagne CT, Diagne MM, Faye M, Faye O, et al. Development, validation and clinical evaluation of a broad-range pan-filovirus RT-qPCR. Journal of Clinical Virology. 2019;**114**:26-31

[26] Nkangu MN, Olatunde OA, Yaya S. The perspective of gender on the Ebola virus using a risk management and population health framework: A scoping review. Infectious Diseases of Poverty. 2017;**6**(1):135

[27] Shorten RJ, Brown CS, Jacobs M, Rattenbury S, Simpson AJ, Mepham S. Diagnostics in Ebola virus disease in resource-rich and resource-limited settings. PLoS Neglected Tropical Diseases. 2016;**10**(10):e0004948

Chapter 6

The Emerging Challenges in Transmission and Detection of Filovirus Infections in Developing Countries

Samuel Okware

Abstract

This chapter reviews the emerging challenges in the transmission and detection of Ebola and Marburg filoviruses since their identification in 1967 and 1976, respectively. Five known highly fatal Ebola species are examined. Ebola outbreaks comprising of 14 EBOV, 7 SUDV, and 4 BDBV infections are reviewed, including the largest West African Ebola outbreak. The ecology of filoviruses and the possible interactions with intermediate hosts and reservoirs is also examined. Evidence that bats are the principal reservoirs of these infections is reviewed. Surveys raise the possibility that other nonhuman primates including dogs may be involved. Challenges on the presumed modes of transmission are discussed with a possibility of droplet and aerosol routes. The discovery of Ebola virus in pigs and its potential impact on the food chain are discussed. The WHO Syndrome Case definition guidelines for diagnosis are examined and shortcomings discussed. However, the early case detection is undermined by the many tropical diseases with similar symptoms. The low positive predictive value for diagnosis based on the antibody antigen assays in outbreaks complicates early isolation and action especially in resource constrained settings. The chapter suggests improvements and areas for further research on the ecology, transmission, and management of filovirus infections.

Keywords: filoviruses, Ebola, Marburg, ecology, reservoirs, transmission, detection

1. Introduction

The filovirus infections are emerging new infections, which pose serious public health threats of global dimensions. This filovirus family comprises mainly of the Ebola virus and the Marburg virus. Some five species of Ebola have been confirmed and includes the Zaire Ebola virus (EBOV), the Sudan subtype (SUDV), the Bundibugyo virus (BDBV), the Tai Forest virus (TAFV), and the Reston virus (RESTV) [1, 2]. Most of the outbreaks have been caused by EBOV and SUDV infections. The TAFV has caused single causality. RESTV is associated with asymptomatic infection among nonhuman primates and pigs [3]. There is yet no known bat hosts for the Sudan, Bundibugyo, or the Tai Forest Ebolavirus.

The Marburg virus was first isolated in 1967 when laboratory workers in Marburg, Germany and Yugoslavia were infected when exposed to imported green monkeys from Uganda [4, 5]. Between 1975 and 1997, a few sporadic cases of Marburgvirus (Marburg virus and the Ravn virus) were reported in South Africa. This was followed in 1980 and in 1987 by sporadic cases in Kenya [1, 4]. Between 1995 and 1999, small outbreaks of Marburg were reported in the Democratic Republic of the Congo. Larger Marburg outbreaks have occurred in the Republic of Congo (1998–2000), Angola (2004–2005), and Uganda (2007–2008) [6, 7]. In 2012, four more similar outbreaks were reported in Uganda and the Democratic Republic of Congo.

The Ebola virus was first identified in 1976 in a major outbreak in 1976. The disease was located in Kikwit near Ebola river in the then northern Zaire [8]. At the same time, a similar outbreak caused by the Sudan subtype also occurred in the current Southern Sudan. Both infections resulted in a high case fatality rate (range 53–89%). Clinical features include high fever, hemorrhagic manifestations, and coagulation defects. Minor outbreaks followed occurring in the Eastern (formerly) Zaire in 1977. Some 34 cases also occurred in Sudan in 1979. There were no further Ebola outbreaks until 1994. From 1994 to 1997, there were a number of outbreaks in DRC, to be followed subsequently by several epidemics between 2000 and 2004 [9]. In 2000, a large outbreak occurred in Gulu Uganda during which 224 cases and 173 deaths were confirmed [10]. In 2007, a novel Bundibugyo Ebola virus caused 116 cases and 39 deaths in Western Uganda [7]. During the same year, a similar outbreak occurred in DRC involving 260 cases with 186 deaths. In several instances, the index case was linked to eating of bats as food [11, 12]. In 2012, three minor outbreaks occurred in Uganda; and one more was reported in the Democratic Republic of the Congo. From 2013 to 2015, the largest Ebola outbreak occurred in West Africa (Guinea, Sierra Leone, and Liberia). It resulted in 28,652 cases and 15,261 deaths affecting heavily the healthcare workers [14]. In May 2018, a new Ebola outbreak erupted in the Equateur Province of the Democratic Republic of the Congo and 50 cases and 25 deaths were reported [13]. In 2019, there is a current ongoing serious outbreak of Ebola in the Eastern Democratic Republic of the Congo on the border with Uganda and over 1000 deaths have so far been reported by September. A single imported case was reported in Western Uganda but was quickly contained. Since 1976, some 25 Ebola outbreaks were reported and comprised of 14 EBOV outbreaks, seven more due to SUDV, and four linked to BDBV infection. In Uganda, some five Ebola outbreaks have been confirmed [15], major one in 2000 and four in 2012.

The aim of this chapter is to review the current knowledge on filoviruses as emerging infections based on published literature with a focus on Ebola and Marburg virus infections and outbreaks. The chapter examines the challenges related to their ecology, transmission, and detection, particularly in developing countries.

2. Role of bats

The natural history of filoviruses remains rudimentary and largely not well understood. The perceived view is that their transmission is a zoonosis linked to wild life, particularly bats. Bats have an economic and ecologic impact on the environment in several ways depending on their feeding habits as insectivorous, frugivorous, or nectarivorous. Bats facilitate plant pollination and the control of insects. Bats are also often eaten in parts of Africa. Falling fruits are often a shared food resource with nonhuman primates and other animals. During the West

African Ebola outbreak, serologic evidence also showed that 31.8% of the dogs were infected, but Ebola like symptoms were not detected in dogs [14]. Studies suggest that nonhuman primates are equally susceptible. An Ebola outbreak occurred among a chimpanzee community in the Tai National Park in Ivory Coast [16] suggesting that they may not be reservoirs. Similar epizootics among other wildlife have also been documented in Gabon [17]. It is possible that Marburg and Ebola persist in hosts that are rare. Recently, a new Ebolavirus called Bombali virus (BOMV) was isolated in house dwelling bats in Sierra Leone raising the possibility of other transmitters [18]. The persistence and resilience of bats and association with most such epidemics remain elusive.

Nonetheless, bats have been recognized as the reservoirs of Ebola. When experimentally inoculated with the Ebola virus, the bats got infected but survived [19]. Surveys have also detected anti-Ebola IgG antibodies in bats [11]. The 2007 outbreak of Marburg virus disease in Kamwenge district in Uganda was associated with a large colony of bats in Kitaka mine. A survey of bats in the cave revealed that 5% of the thousands of fruit bats in the mine were harboring the Marburg virus [20]. The presence of Ebola and Marburg virus antibodies in fruit bats [9] has also been confirmed. Antibodies against ZEBOV and RESTV have also been detected from bats in Indonesia, China, and Bangladesh [21, 22]. Transmission risks could be increased during mating, birthing, or in group migration. These events are seasonal. Understanding their ecology and habits provides critical knowledge on perceived risks associated with seasonality. Indeed some studies have revealed that high transmission is associated with birthing [23].

Studies on cross immunity and reactivity amidst circulating filovirus antibodies in bats could evaluate the extent of their asymptomatic status. Studies should be done to determine the routes of infection and to assess the viral load in tissues of bats and related sources of infection. Little is known about the natural long term immunological, pathological, and clinical responses to filovirus infection in bats. Studies on immunological responses in bats in their natural settings are required to determine the role of bats in harboring and sustaining infection. The apparent observed asymptomatic infection despite the viremia and apparent immunity in bats needs long-term investigation. There are still gaps in identifying routes of viral shedding, seasonality, other animal and probably insect reservoirs in the ecology of these viruses. The observed relationships and potential implications need further exploration of the ecology of the filoviruses in their natural hosts.

The geographical range of bats able to be hosts filoviruses is reported to be very extensive and geographically very broad. For instance, bats in the Iberian Peninsula were reported to have died of viral pneumonia in a cave in Northern Spain (Cueva del Lloviu). The cause was reported to be due to a new filovirus named Lloviu virus [24]. There are over 1200 species of bats identified globally, of which only a few have been screened for filoviruses [21].

3. Challenges in transmission

Epidemiological evidence suggests that the major mode of transmission for Ebola and Marburg infections is through direct contact with infected blood or body fluids. Nonsterile needles and administration of blood equally pose a potential risks especially in low resource settings. Thus, healthcare workers and bed side healthcare givers of patients are exposed to exceptional nosocomial risks [7, 25, 26]. Long-term persistence of Ebola in semen (up to 179 days) has been shown post recovery. There are also reports of Ebola transmission occurring through breast milk of asymptomatic individuals during the West Africa outbreak. These observations underscore the possible transmission through breast feeding and sexual contact with survivors of infection [27, 28]. Large scale outbreaks of Marburg virus have been linked to mines and caves [6, 20, 29] suggesting the possibility of other routes of spread. In such circumstances, it is not clear whether the routes of infection are via droplets, bat excreta, or even the aerosol route. Aerosols are generated from the respiratory tract through coughing, breathing, and talking and could cause droplet or airborne spread of infection. This could be a rare but important mode of spread of infection. However, data on this concept are small and the role of aerosol route emerging as a possibility needs to be examined. In addition, the role of fomites in amplifying transmission and spread of the infection needs investigation. Additional studies are required to segregate the significance of aerosol and droplet transmission. Ebola virus has been isolated from saliva and pulmonary alveoli in experimental animals; thus, making a case for the droplet transmission. Cough and pneumonitis is a symptom of both Ebola and Marburg filovirus disease and further strengthens the infection potential via this route as already demonstrated and suggested by RESTV experiments with pigs and monkeys. However, it is possible that some patients infected with the EBOV West African Strain (Makoma) have higher viral loads and infectivity [14]. Further studies are required to determine the dynamics and mechanisms for such transmission through indirect contact. There are also reports that pigs when infected with Ebola virus can infect the cynomolgus macaques in the absence of direct contact. Animal to animal studies have also demonstrated fatal infection through inhalation of aerosol and droplets in caged monkeys. Similar other animal studies have demonstrated the transmission of Ebola like disease in inoculated monkeys [30].

Nonetheless, isolation of patients remains the basis for containing the further spread of infection [31]. However, this has not always been perfect in low resource settings. In Uganda, it has been reported that 64% of the 31 infected healthcare workers got infection after the provision of personal protection measures and the establishment of isolation facilities [15]. The inadequacy of training on use of personal protection material was postulated as a contributing factor. False assurance and complacency that the general wards were safe could have compromised protection. Other victims included support staff like ambulance drivers felt a false sense of security since they were not working in the isolation wards. Some of the victims worked exclusively in general wards or were support staff like ambulance drivers and cleaners. However, there may be other host factors including societal obstacles such as special attachment when caring for dear relatives, which accentuated vulnerability to infection.

4. Challenges in clinical detection

Early detection remains vital for prompt action for the control of filoviruses in emergencies. Clinical assessment based on symptoms assisted by the laboratory is usually applied to identify and manage cases of Ebola of Marburg Virus diseases. The WHO case definition guideline is used to categorize “alert,” “suspected,” “probable,” or “confirmed” cases. The typical clinical features consist of high fever of sudden onset in a contact. This is usually associated with cough, diarrhea, and bleeding manifestations and the patient quickly dies within days due to shock and multi organ failure. The challenge, however, is the presence of many tropical diseases that mimic this syndrome. Malaria for instance is endemic in Equatorial Africa, where most outbreaks occur. The sensitivity and specificity of the clinical case definition as well as its positive predictive value is largely unknown from outbreak to the other. Confirmation based on laboratory ELISA and antigen tests equally has a very low positive predictive value of less than 50% [15]. This may be compounded further by a significant presence of Ebola and Marburg IgG antibodies among asymptomatic individuals in the rain forests of Central Africa. Sero-surveys in some countries in Equatorial Africa reveal that the Ebola virus IgG prevalence was 5.3% while for Marburg it was 2.4%. The pigmy population had a significantly higher IgG prevalence of 7.02% [32]. An even high ZEBOV specific seroprevalence of 19.4% was found near the rain forests in the Demographic Republic of the Congo [33]. Surveys in identified populations in Equatorial Africa have revealed significant prevalence of Ebola IgG antibodies among asymptomatic individuals [9, 33–35]. This suggests some cross-reactions or past mild infection with diverse filoviruses. The observation probably suggests frequent contact between human and less virulent strains. Thus, the management of outbreaks including the identification and isolation, discharge and care has real limitations. Therefore, it is desirable to concurrently determine the sensitivity and the specificity of these detection methods during ongoing outbreaks and refine the case definition. More sensitive noninventive methods of detection to support surveys in wildlife would support our understanding of the natural course of filovirus illness.

5. Challenges to food security

Food security is an issue to consider in view of the reported filovirus infection in pigs and bats. In some parts of Africa, bats are often eaten and fruits are a shared food source with wild animals. It has been reported that the Ebola virus has been found in frugivorous bats. These bats if they come into close contact with humans through the fruits such as coconuts, a shared food source, could pose a potential danger. Marburgvirus has also been isolated from orangutan primates in Indonesia [36]. Isolates of Ebola virus from wild apes also reveal genetic lineage and recombinants [37]. This interface makes it possible for the infection to be acquired from these suspected intermediate hosts or reservoirs. Infection to susceptible humans through the primary or intermediate reservoirs such as chimpanzees, pigs, and duikers or directly through the food source may contaminate the food chain and propagate the infection. The role of other suspected reservoirs including arthropod vectors, rodents, and plants [19, 38] while unlikely is unknown and should be studied.

6. Conclusion

Filoviruses are emerging infections that present considerable challenges in understanding their elusive ecology, transmission, and reservoirs particularly bats. Direct contact with infected blood and body fluids remains the major mode of transmission of both viruses. The discovery of new subtypes of Ebola and other viruses shows increasing diversity in the evolution of these viruses. The ecology and the evolving dynamics of these viruses need to be examined to identify those other related hosts and viruses. While it is generally accepted that the filoviruses are transmitted through direct contact, there is evidence that respiratory transmission through aerosols and droplets can be considered in massive outbreaks. While we also know that transmission does not place before symptoms emerge, additional data should refine the exact onset of infectiousness. The virus may be shed for some months post recovery through semen and breast milk among survivors.

The possible amplification of transmission by domestic or wild animals during the massive West African outbreak sheds some light on the role of such animal to human interface. The possibility of Ebola and Marburg entering the food chain and compromising safety should be assessed especially in pork and pork products. Case detection of index cases in emergencies presents a real challenge in low resource settings. The case definition of diagnosis and algorithms for management should be refined and validated regularly to improve on the positive predictive value of screening tests.

A global strategy for surveillance of filoviruses is required for a coordinated worldwide strategy and response that will mitigate the global impact of future outbreaks. Disease management needs evidence from ecological studies and prevention and control strategies should adopt One Health concept, which integrates animal and human health interventions to support early detection, surveillance, prevention, and control.

Author details

Samuel Okware
Uganda National Health Research Organisation, Entebbe, Uganda

*Address all correspondence to: okwares@gmail.com

References

[1] Peters CJ. Filovirues as emerging pathogens. Seminars in Virology. 1994;**5**:147-154

[2] Shirode L. Ebola virus disease: A review on epidemiology, pathogenesis, transmission and treatment. World Journal of Pharmaceutical Research. 2015;**4**:819-826

[3] Smith DH, Johnson BK, Isaacson M, Swanapoel R, Johnson KM, Killey M, et al. Marburg_Marburg-virus disease in Kenya. Lancet. 1982;**1**(8276):816-820

[4] Smith DH et al. Marburg-virus disease in Kenya. Lancet. 1982;**1**(8276):816-820

[5] Henssen W. In: Martin GA, Siegert R, editors. Epidemiology of Marburg Virus Disease. Springer Verlag; 1971. pp. 161-165

[6] Brauburger K. Forty five years of Marburg virus research. Viruses. 2012;**4**:1878-1927

[7] Wamala JF et al. Ebola hemorrhagic fever associated with novel virus strain, Uganda, 2007-2008. Emerging Infectious Diseases. 2010;**16**(7):1087-1092

[8] Heymann DL et al. Ebola hemorrhagic fever: Tandala, Zaire, 1977-1978. The Journal of Infectious Diseases. 1980;**142**(3):372-376

[9] Pourrut X et al. Large serological survey showing cocirculation of Ebola and Marburg viruses in Gabonese bat populations, and a high seroprevalence of both viruses in *Rousettus aegyptiacus*. BMC Infectious Diseases. 2009;**9**:159

[10] Okware SI et al. An outbreak of Ebola in Uganda. Tropical Medicine & International Health. 2002;7(12):1068-1075

[11] Leroy EM et al. Fruit bats as reservoirs of Ebola virus. Nature. 2005;**438**(7068):575-576

[12] Leroy E. Human Ebola outbreak resulting from direct exposure to fruit bats in Luebo, Democratic Republic of the Congo, 2007. Vector-Borne and Zoonotic Diseases. 2009;**9**:723-728

[13] Barry A et al. Ebola_Outbreak of Ebola virus disease in the Democratic Republic of the Congo, April–May, 2018: An epidemiological study. The Lancet. 2018;**392**(10143):213-221

[14] Osterholm MT, Moore KA, Gostin LO. Public health in the age of ebola in West Africa. JAMA Internal Medicine. 2015;**175**(1):7-8

[15] Okware S. Three Outbreaks of Ebola in Uganda, in BORA (Bergen Office of Reseach Archives). 2015. p. 37

[16] Formenty PB. Ebla virus outbreak among wild chimpanzees living in a rain forest of cote d'Ivoire. The Journal of Infectious Diseases. 1999;**179**(S1):S120-S126

[17] Georges AJ et al. Ebola hemorrhagic fever outbreaks in Gabon, 1994-1997: Epidemiologic and health control issues. The Journal of Infectious Diseases. 1999;**179**(Suppl 1):S65-S75

[18] Goldstein T, Anthony SJ, Gbakima A, Bird BH, Bangura J, Tremeau-Bravard A, et al. The discovery of Bombali virus adds further support for bats as hosts of ebolaviruses. Nature Microbiology. 2018;**3**(10):1084-1089

[19] Swanepoel R. Studies of reservoir hosts for Marburg virus. Emerging Infectious Diseases. 2007;**13**:1847-1851

[20] Towner JS et al. Isolation of genetically diverse Marburg viruses

from Egyptian fruit bats. PLoS Pathogens. 2009;**5**(7):e1000536

[21] Olival KJ. Ebolavirus antibodies in fruit bats, Bangladesh. Emerging Infectious Diseases. 2013;**19**:270-273

[22] Yuan JF. Serological evedence of Ebola virus infection in bats, China. Virology Journal. 2012;**9**. DOI: 10.1186/1743-422X-9-236

[23] Amman BR. Seasonal pulses of Marburg virus circulationin juvenile Rousettus aegyptiacus bats coincide with periods of increased risk of human infection. PLoS Pathogens. 2012;**8**. DOI: 10.1371/journal.ppat.1002877

[24] Negredo A. Discory of an ebolavirus-like filovirus in Europe. PLoS Pathogens. 2011;**7**:e1002304. DOI: 10.1371/journal.ppat.1002304

[25] MacNeil A et al. Proportion of deaths and clinical features in Bundibugyo Ebola virus infection, Uganda. Emerging Infectious Diseases. 2010;**16**(12):1969-1972

[26] CDC. Infection Control for Viral Haemorrhagic Fevers in the African Health Care Setting, 1-198. Geneva: WHO; 1998

[27] Sisokko D. Ebola virus persistence in breast milk after no reported illness: A likely source of virus transmission from mother to child. Clinical Infectious Diseases. 2017;**2017**:23

[28] Mate SE, Kugelman JR, Nyenswah TG, et al. Molecular evidence of sexual transmission of ebola virus. New England Journal of Medicine. 2015;**25**(373):373

[29] Bausch D. Marburg haemorrhagic fever associated with multiple genetic lineages of virus. The New England Journal of Medicine. 2006;**355**(9):909-919

[30] Weingartl H. Transmission of Ebola virus from pigs to non-human primates. Scientific Reports. 2012. DOI: 10.1038/srep00811

[31] WHO. Overview of the COMBI Planning Steps in Outbreak Communication. Geneva: WHO; 2012

[32] Gonzalez JP et al. Ebola and Marburg virus antibody prevalence in selected populations of the Central African Republic. Microbes and Infection. 2000;**2**(1):39-44

[33] Becquart P et al. High prevalence of both humoral and cellular immunity to Zaire ebolavirus among rural populations in Gabon. PLoS One. 2010;**5**(2):e9126

[34] Busico KM et al. Prevalence of IgG antibodies to Ebola virus in individuals during an Ebola outbreak, Democratic Republic of the Congo, 1995. The Journal of Infectious Diseases. 1999;**179**(Suppl 1):S102-S107

[35] Kankya C, Nabadda D, Kabonesa C, Nyakarahuka L, Muleme J, Okware S, et al. Social dynamics of ebola virus disease: A case of Bundibugyo District, Uganda. Health. 2019;**11**(1):90297. DOI: 10.4236/health.2019.111011

[36] Nidom CA. Serological evidence of Ebola virus infection in Indonesian orangutans. PLOS One. 2012;**7**:e40740. DOI: 10.1371/journal.pone.0040740

[37] Wittmann TJ. Isolates of Zaire ebolavirus from wild apes reveal genetic lineageand recombinants. Proceedings of the National Academy of Sciences of the United States of America. 2007;**104**:17123-17127

[38] Germain M. Collection of mammals and athropods duringthe epidemic of haemorrhagic fever in Zaire. In: Pattyn SR, editor. Ebola Haemorrhagic Fever. New York, NY, USA: Elsevier; 1978. pp. 185-189